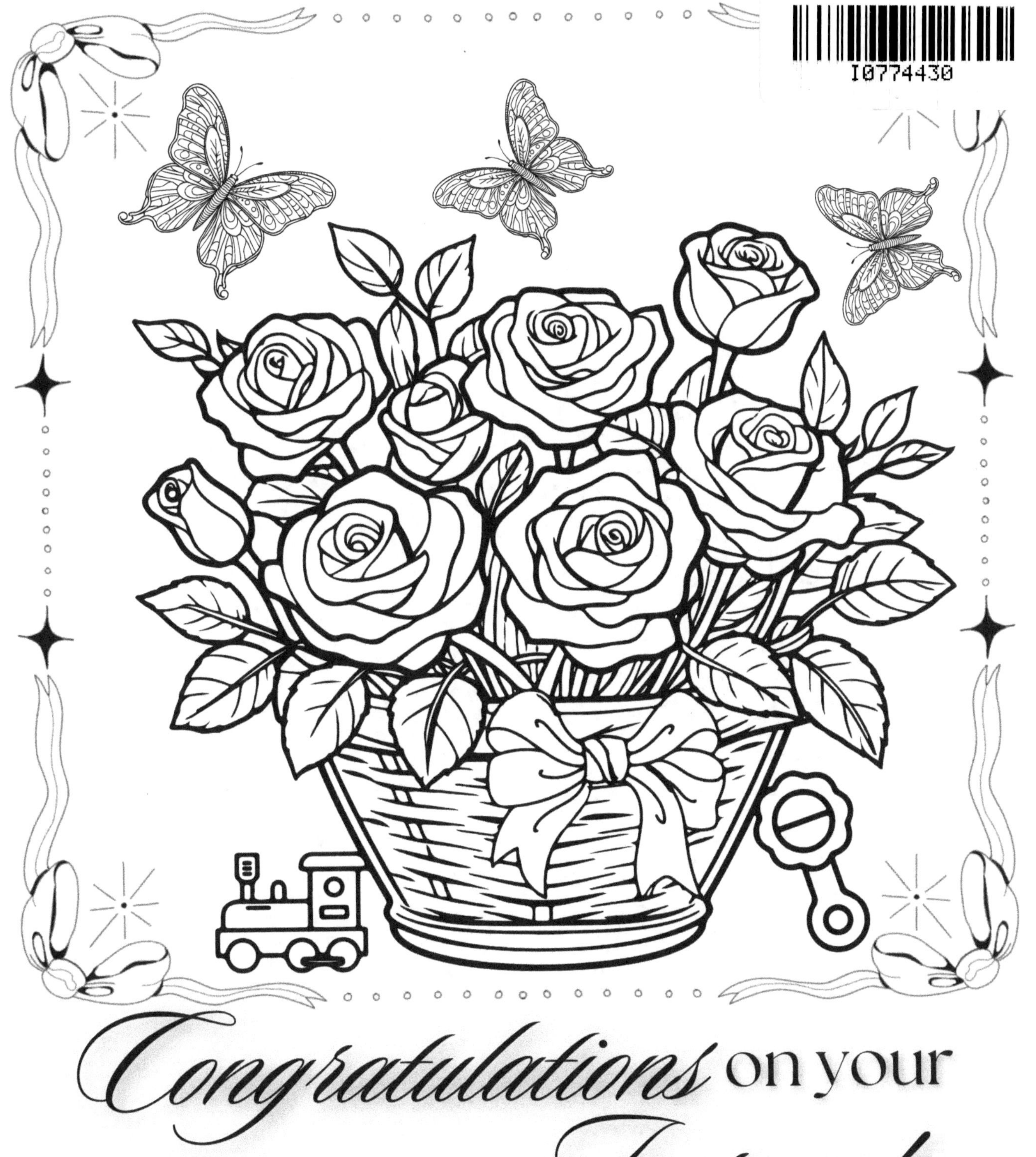

Congratulations on your pregnancy Journey!

WITH WARMEST WISHES,
KB KLINSUKONT

*Dear friend,
remember to take breaks often
and find a comfortable position
to avoid fatigue.*

*Choose safe, non-toxic colors
for your little one.*

*Enjoy the coloring process and relax,
don't pressure yourself.*

I'm always here to support you!

"In the first trimester, your baby is developing rapidly
from an embryo to forming essential organs.
It's an exciting time as you start to notice little changes."

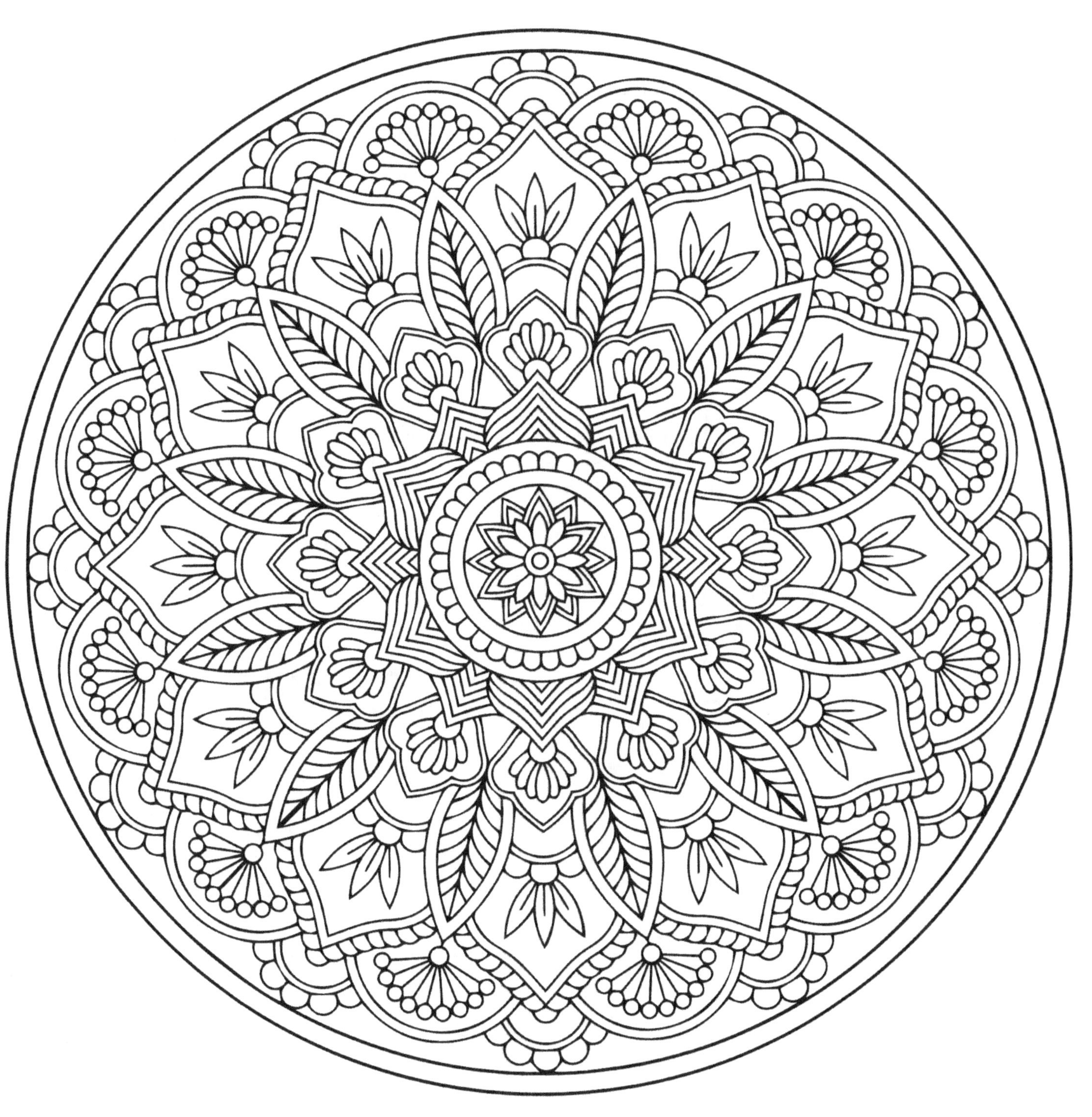

"Welcome to this beautiful journey,
one step at a time"

Growing Together

"You're creating a new life!
Be proud of every step in this amazing journey."

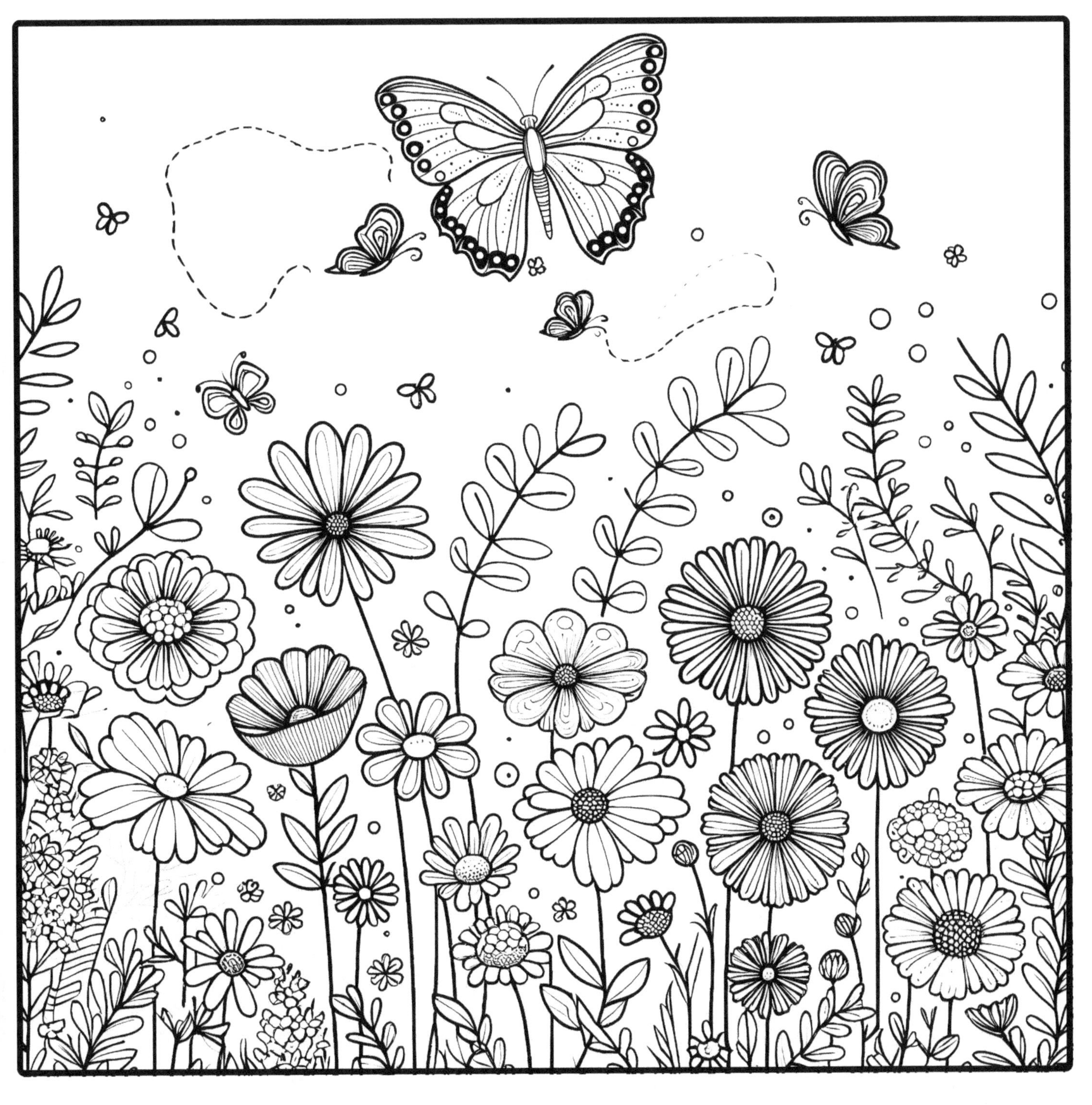

"Just like these flowers,
you're blooming beautifully."

Growing Together

"Coloring and crafting can lift your spirits.
It's like a mini-vacation for your mind!"

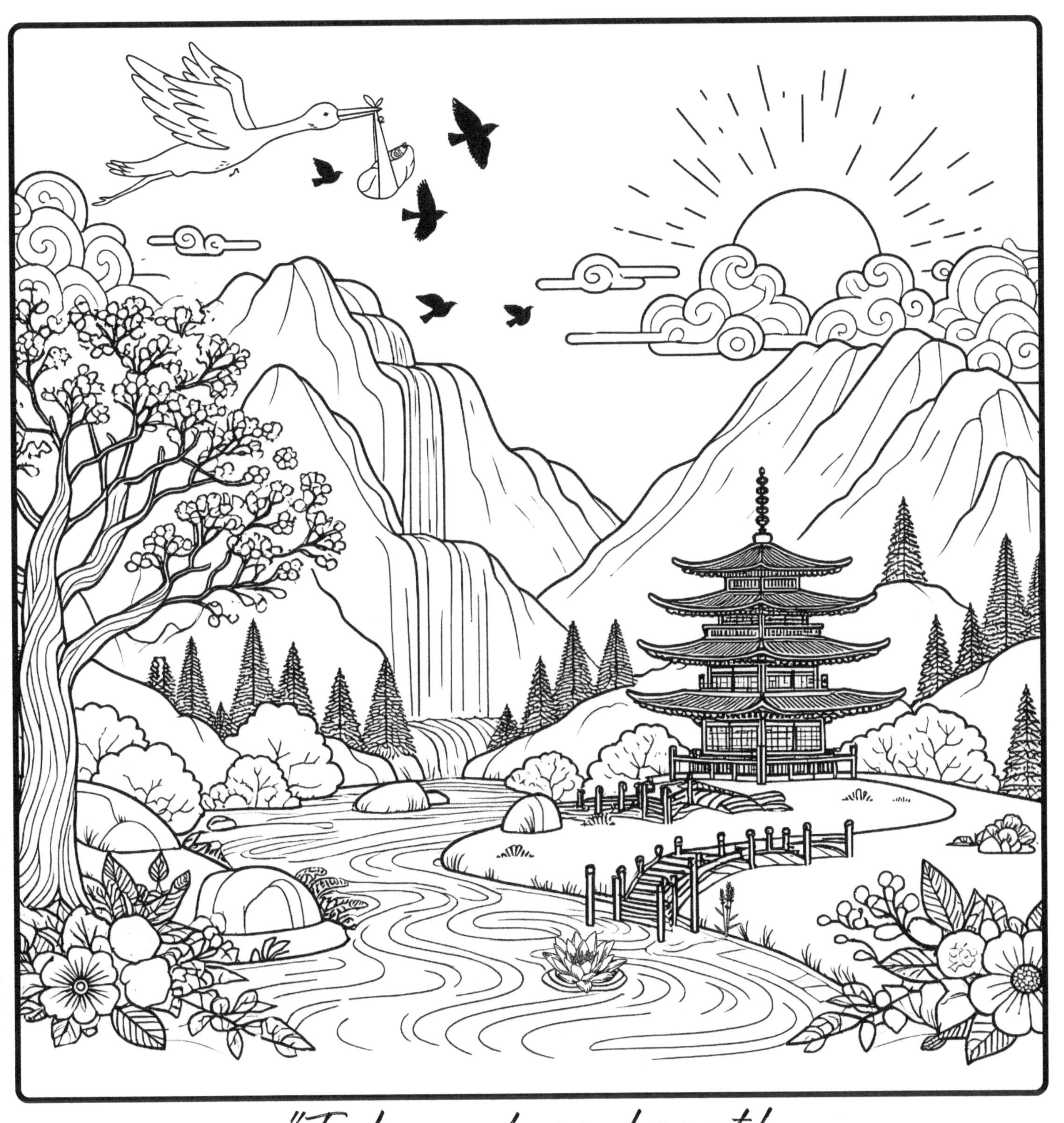

"Take a deep breath,
you're doing amazing, mama"

Growing Together

"In the first trimester,
your baby is growing rapidly from a tiny seed into a little wonder.
It's like a magical secret garden inside you!"

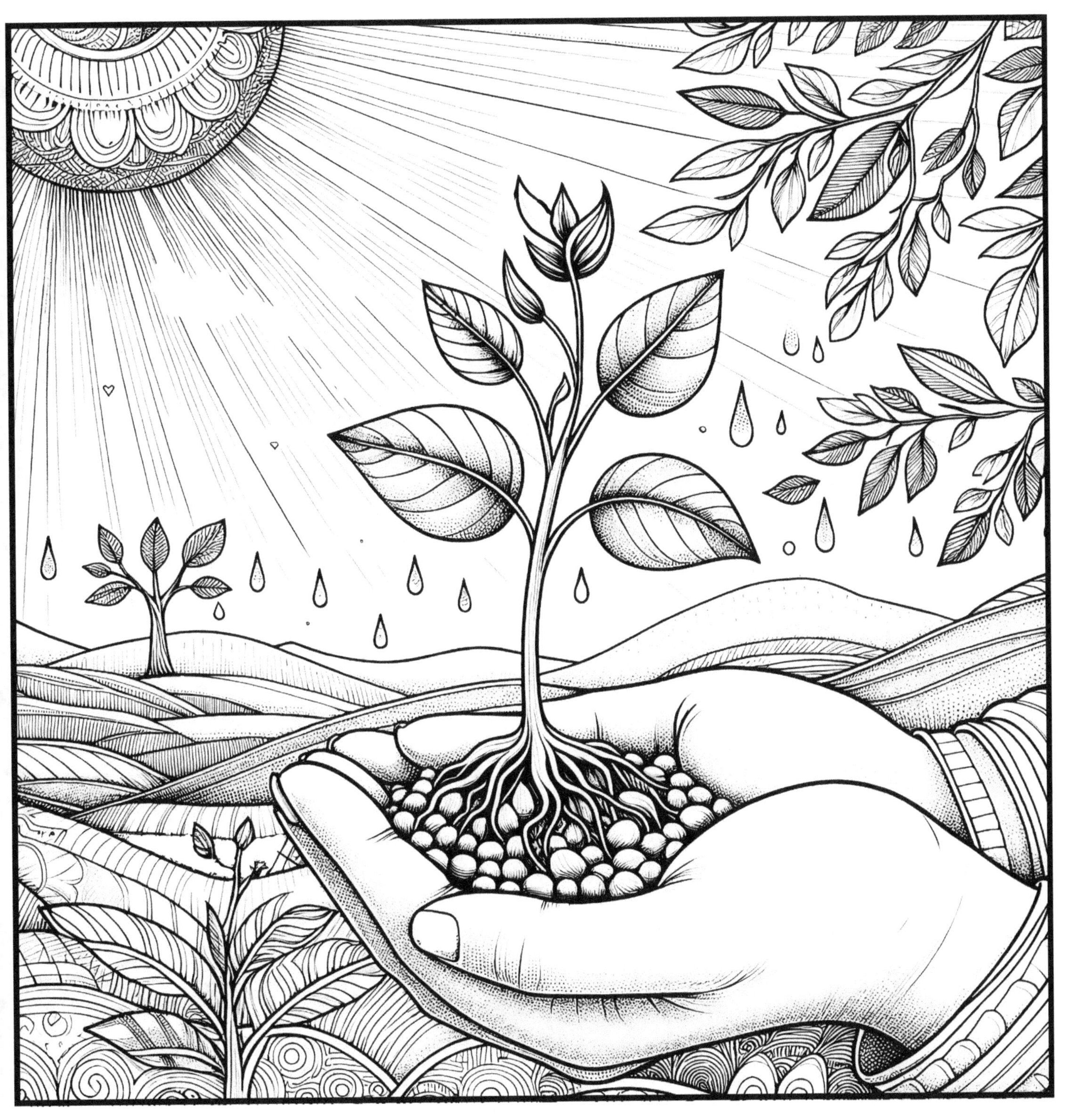

"From tiny seeds, big things grow.
You're nurturing a miracle"

Growing
Together

"Creating a cozy home for your baby
is like building a nest of love and warmth."

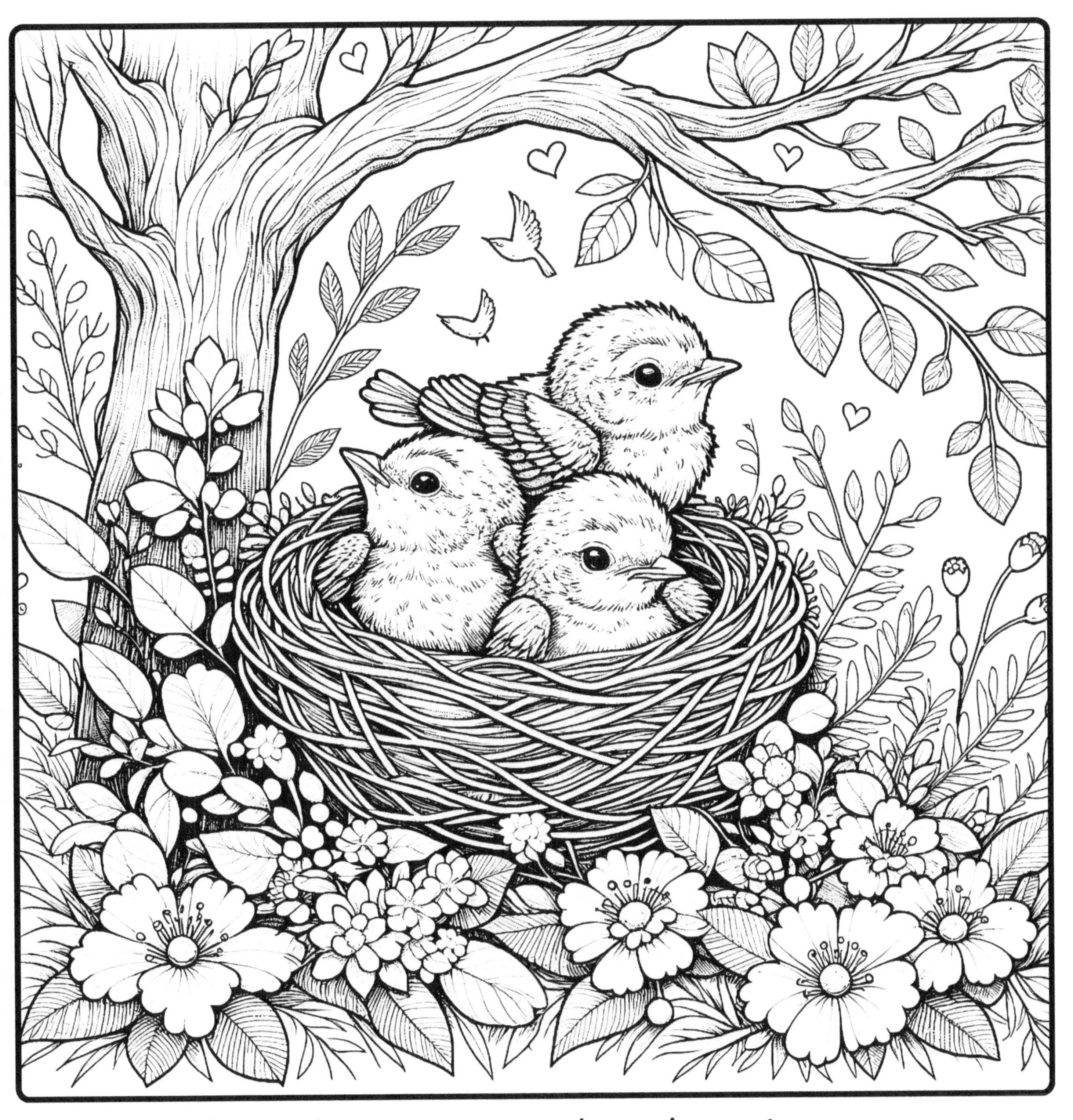

*"Little moments, big love.
Cherish every single one"*

Growing
Together

"Relax and take it easy.
You and your baby deserve all the love and care."

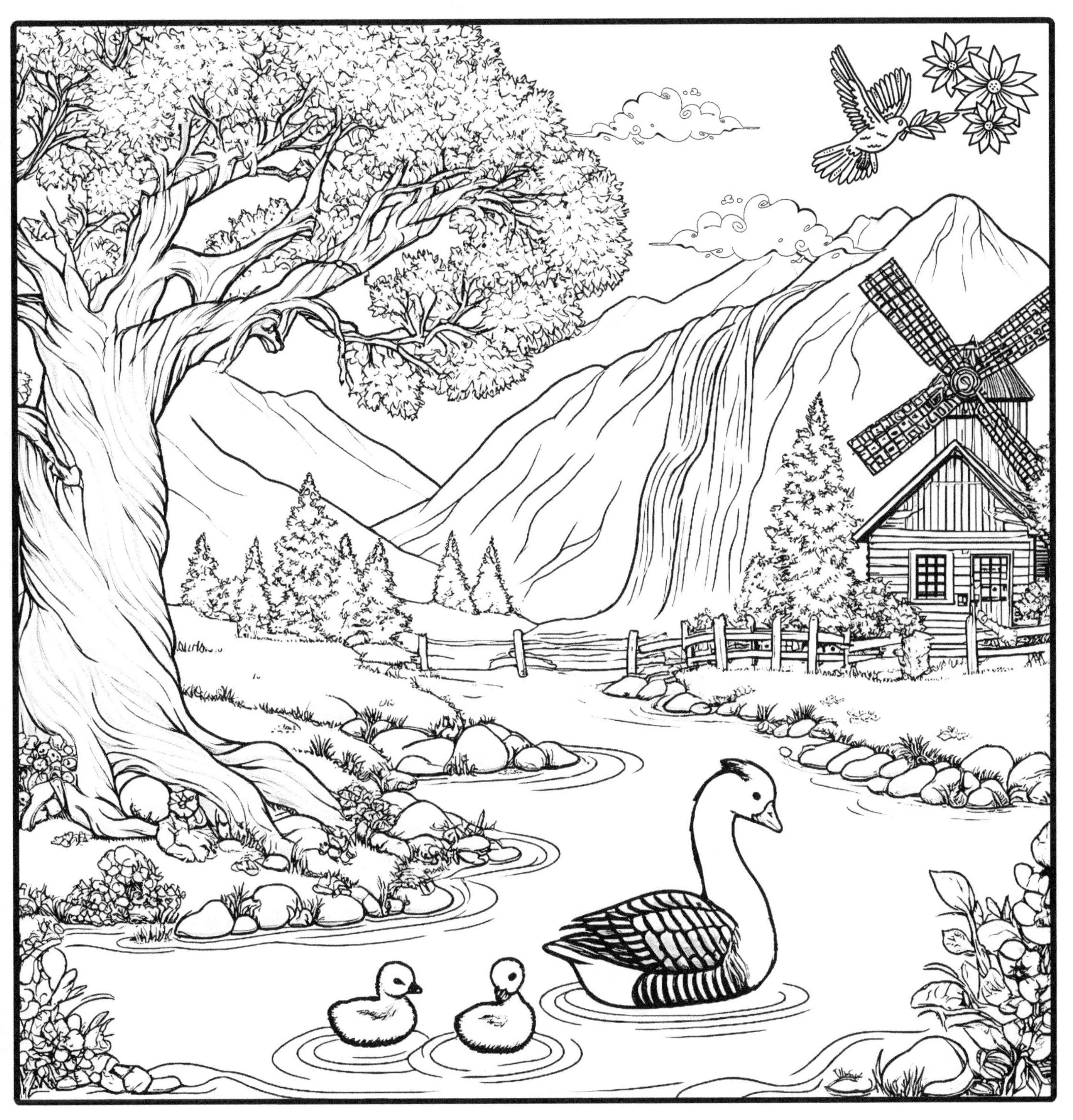

"Find peace in the beauty around you."

Growing Together

"Surround yourself with love and positivity.
It's like building a warm nest for your baby."

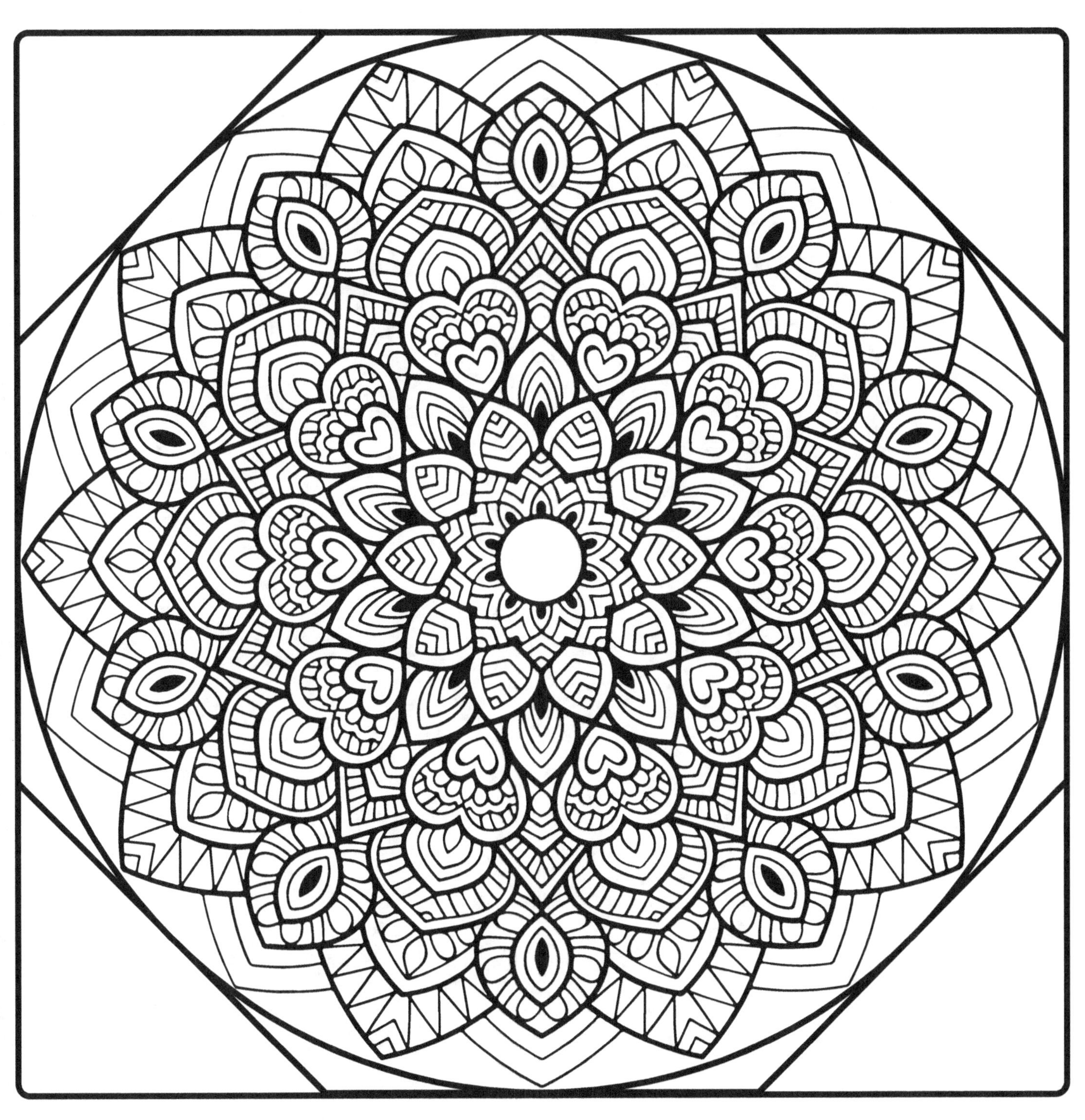

*"Calm your mind,
one stroke at a time"*

Growing Together

"Look at the world with positive eyes.
Happiness is all around you."

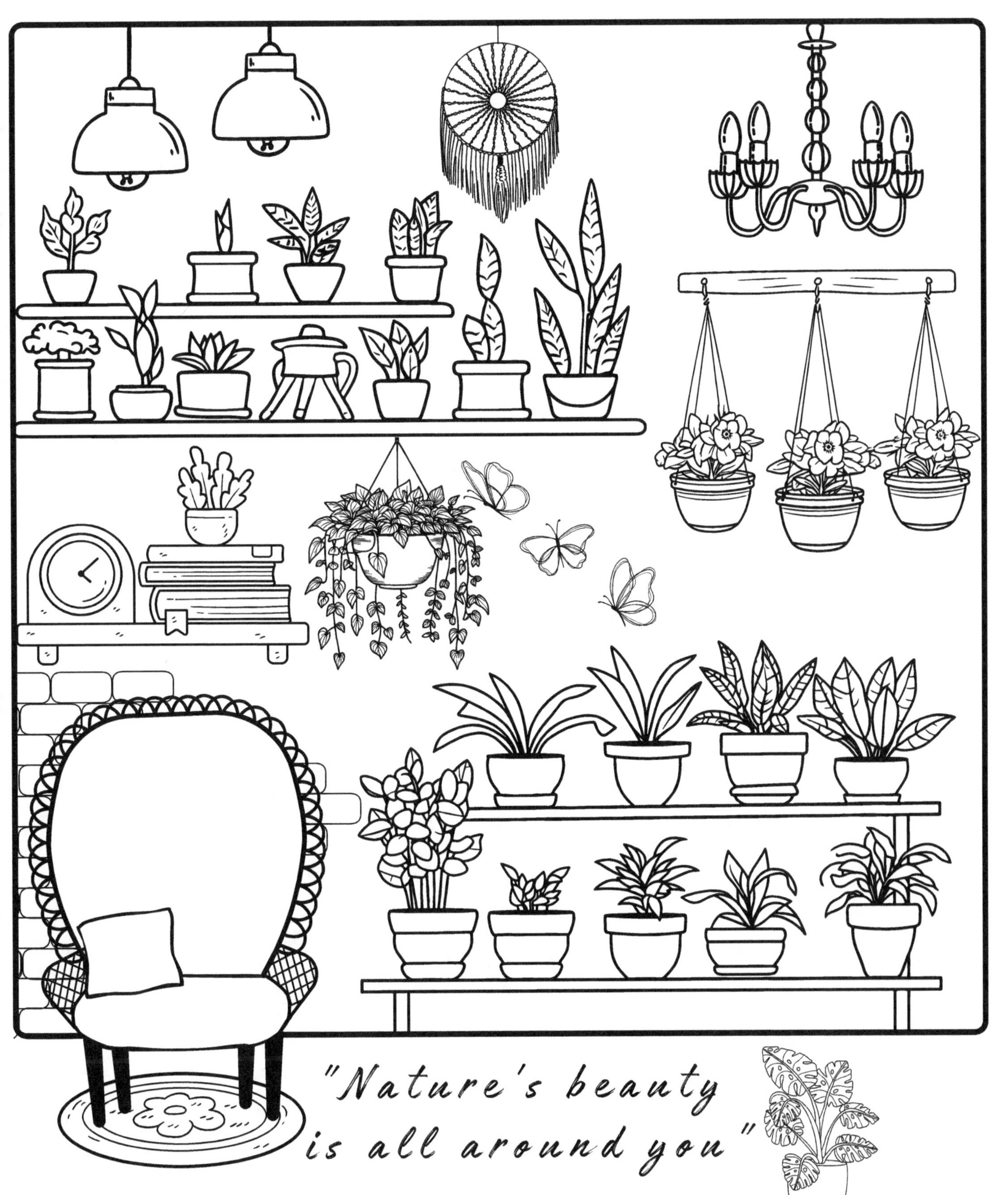
"Nature's beauty
is all around you"

Growing
Together

"Your love is the best nourishment for your baby.
Let your heart lead the way."

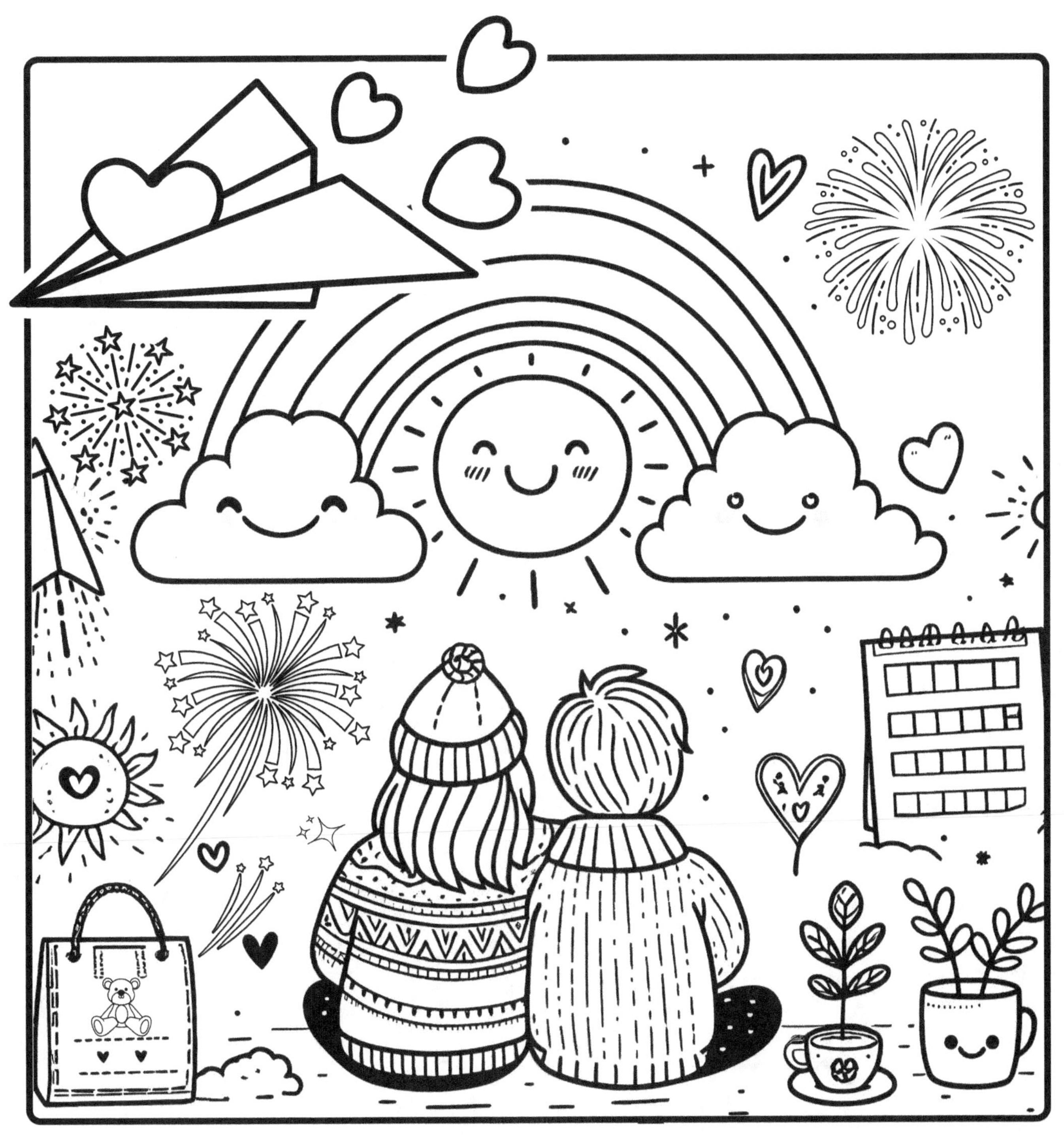

"Bright days are ahead."

Growing Together

"Embrace the changes and look forward to the journey ahead.
Every moment is special."

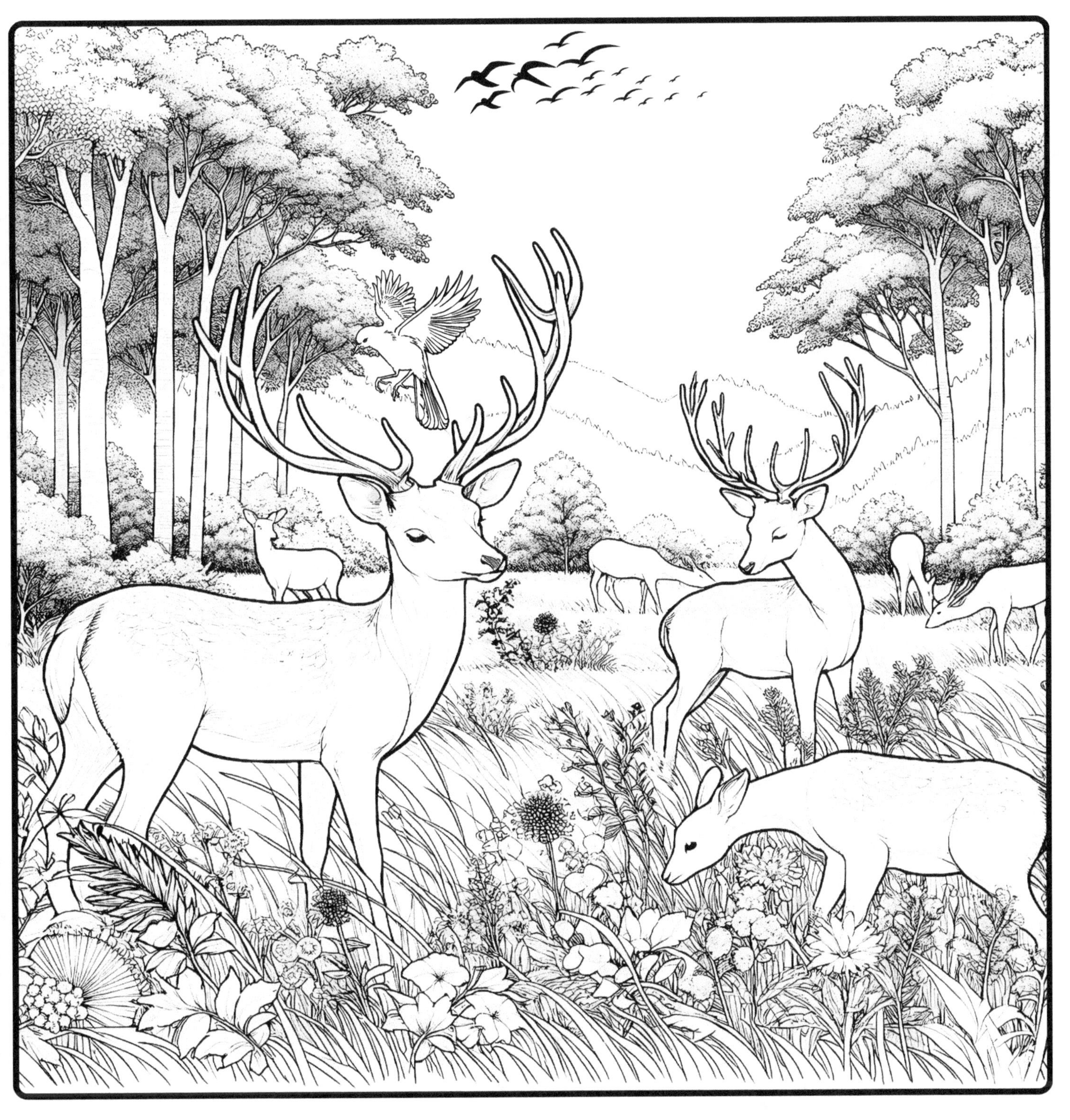

"*Embrace the beauty
of the simple moments.*"

Growing Together

"Bonding with your baby starts now.
Talk to them, sing to them, and share your love."

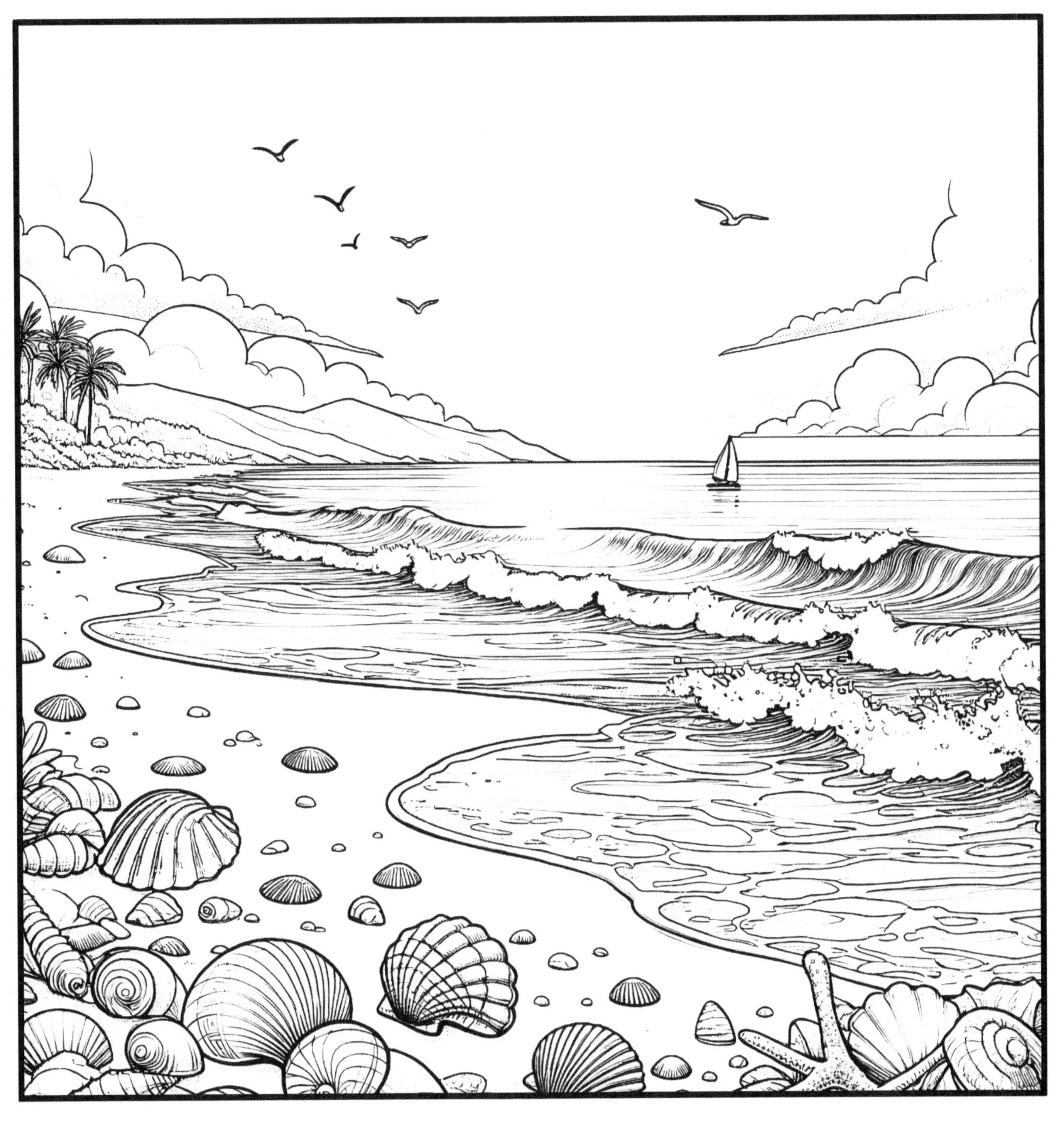

"Let the waves
wash your worries away."

Growing
Together

"Preparing for your baby also means taking care of yourself.
You are important too!"

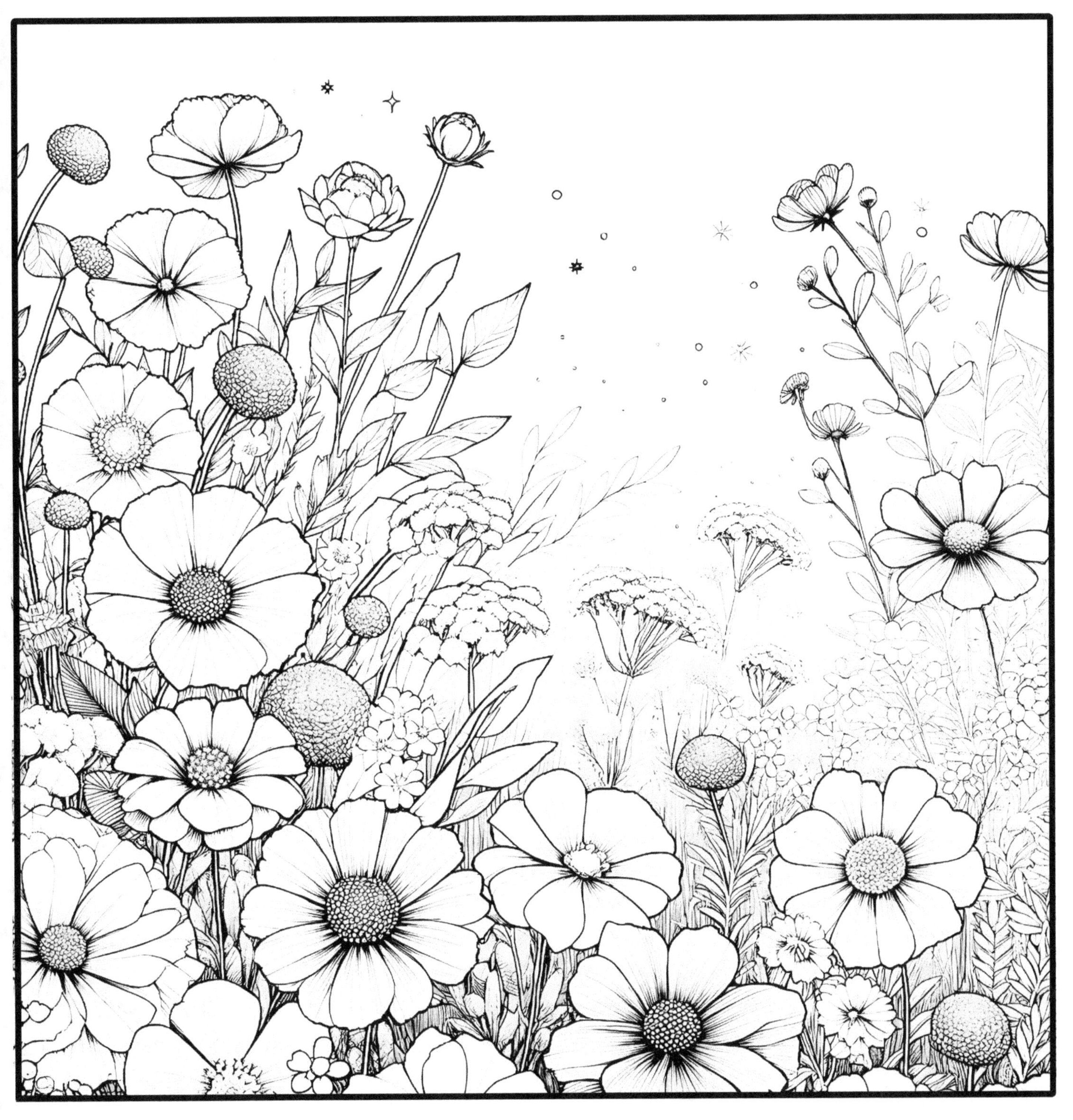

"You are growing and glowing every day."

Growing Together

"Your body is adjusting and producing essential hormones
for your baby's growth. You might feel a bit tired,
but you're doing an amazing job!"

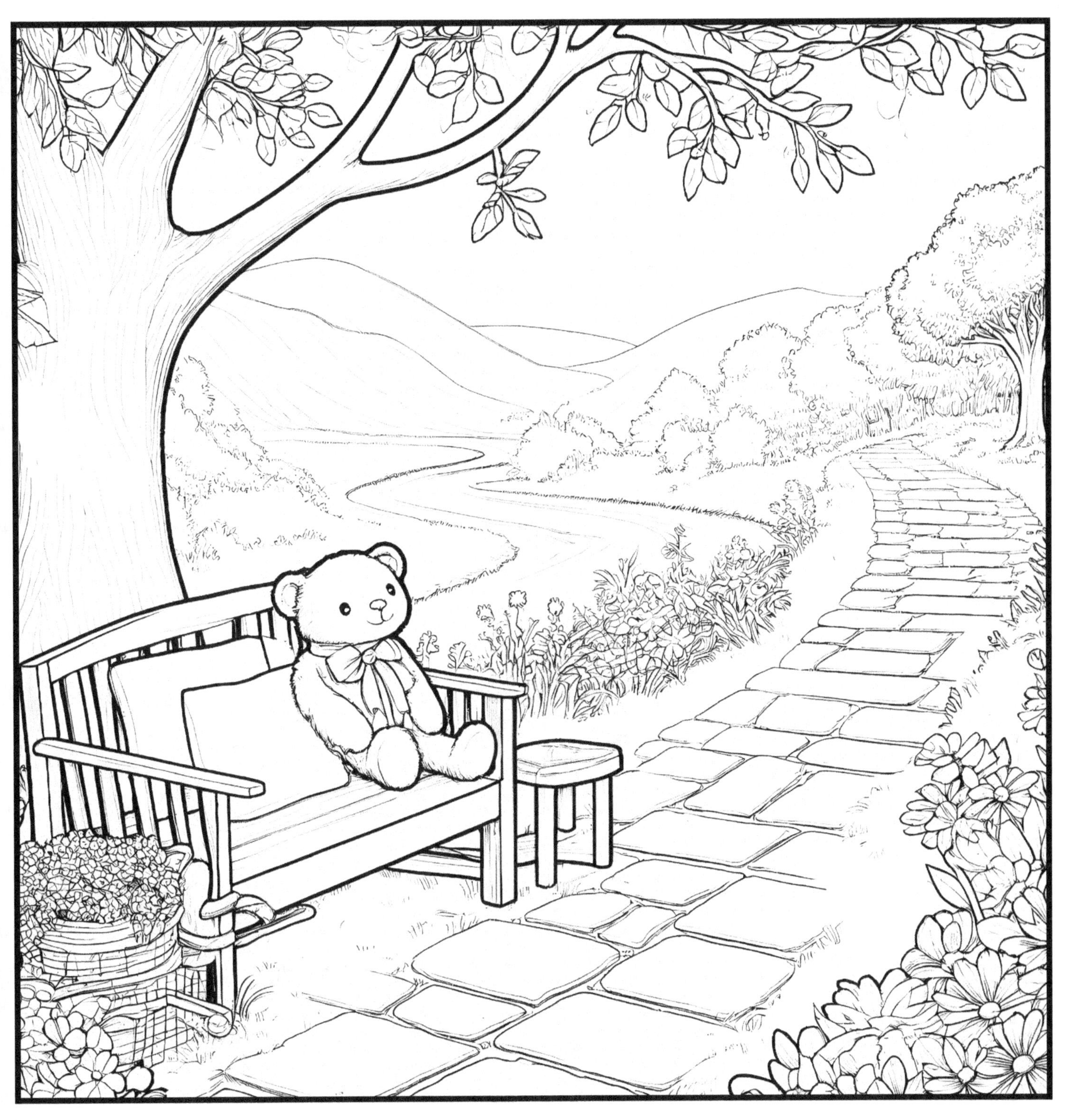

"Trust the journey,
trust yourself."

Growing
Together

"Nature has a calming effect.
A stroll in the garden can fill you with positive energy."

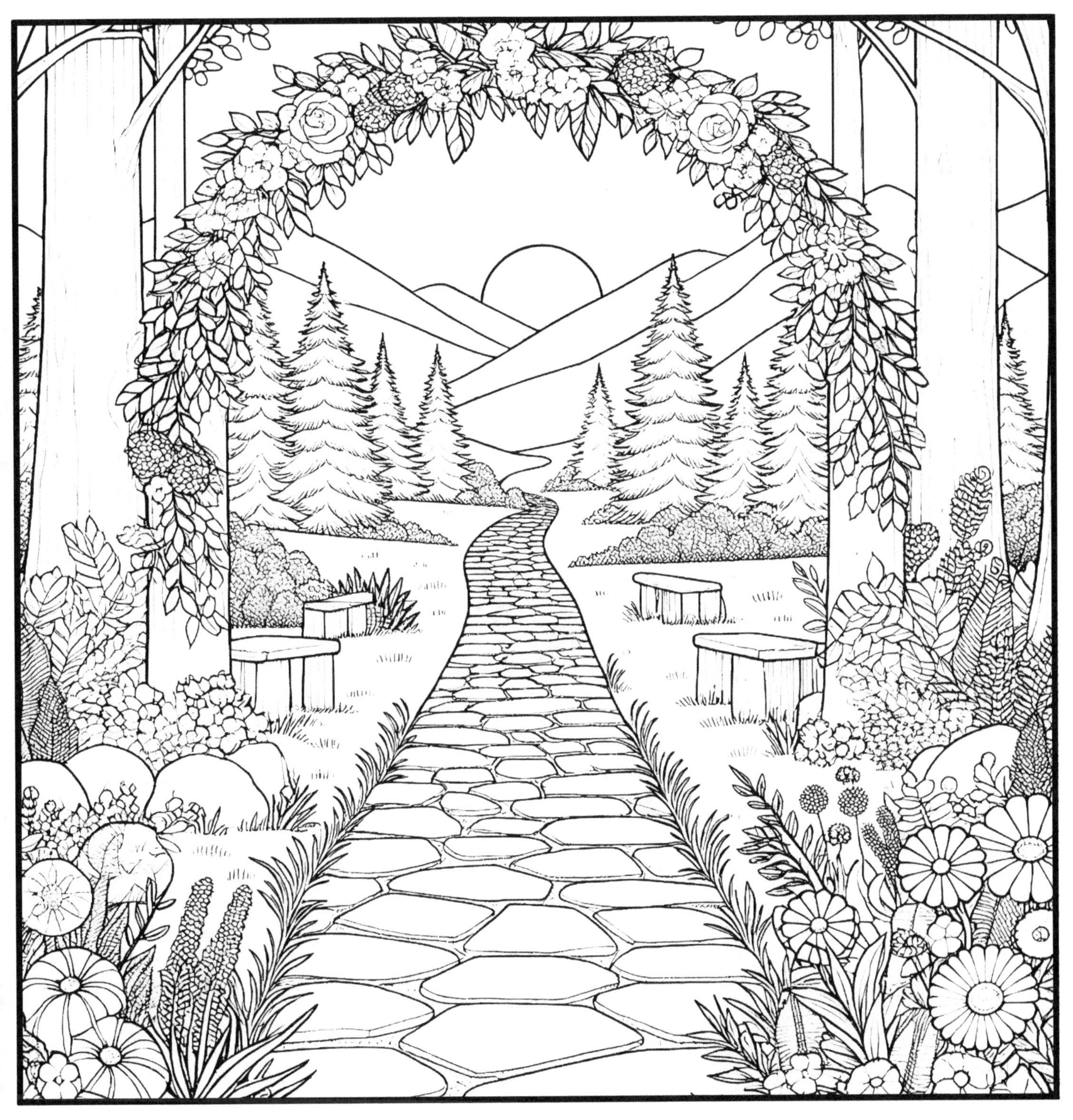

"Every step you take brings you closer
to your little miracle."

Growing Together

"Take time for yourself.
A relaxed and happy mom is the best gift for your baby."

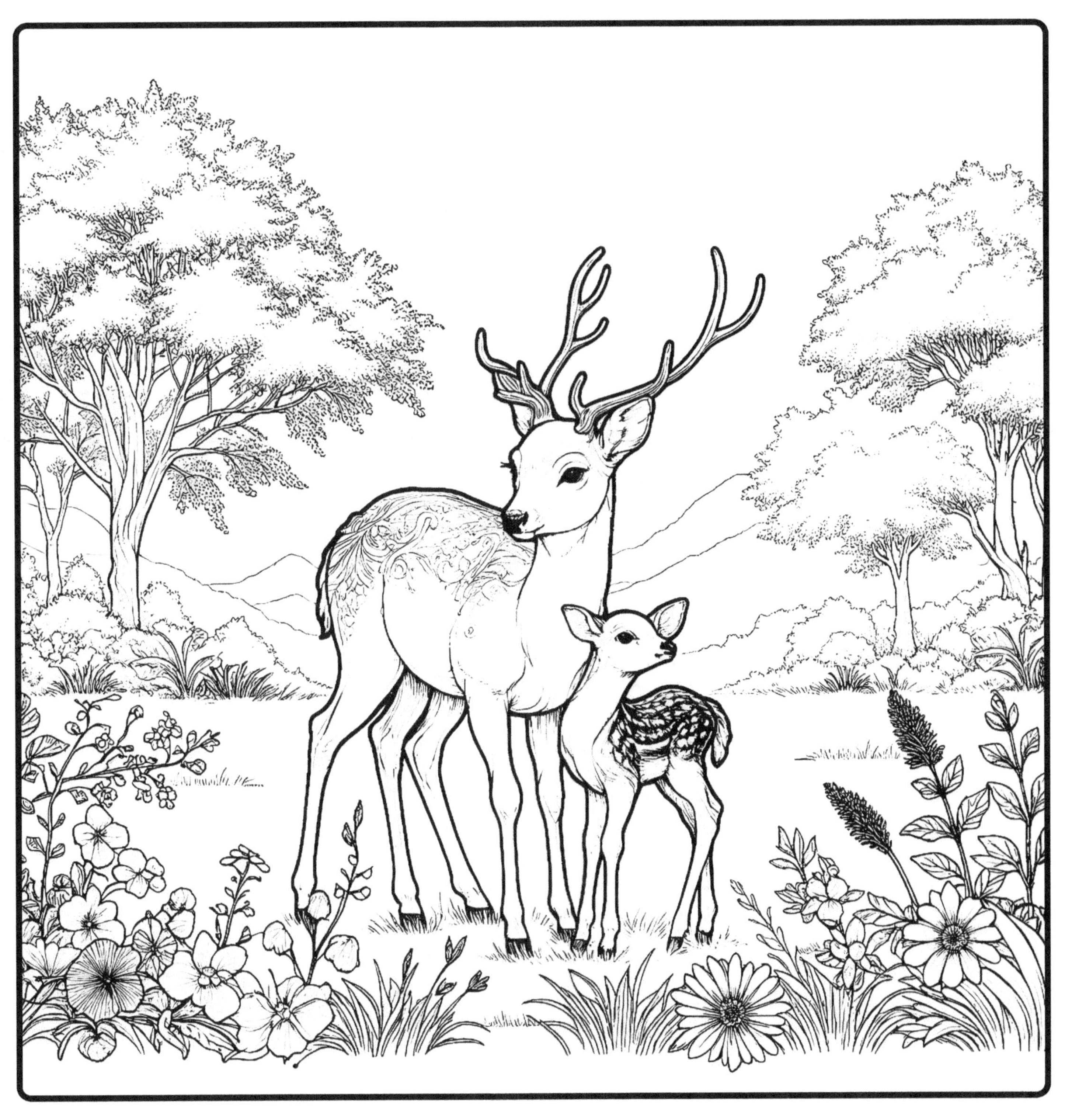

*"Your strength and love
are boundless."*

Growing Together

"Each day brings new experiences and joys.
Savor every moment of this journey."

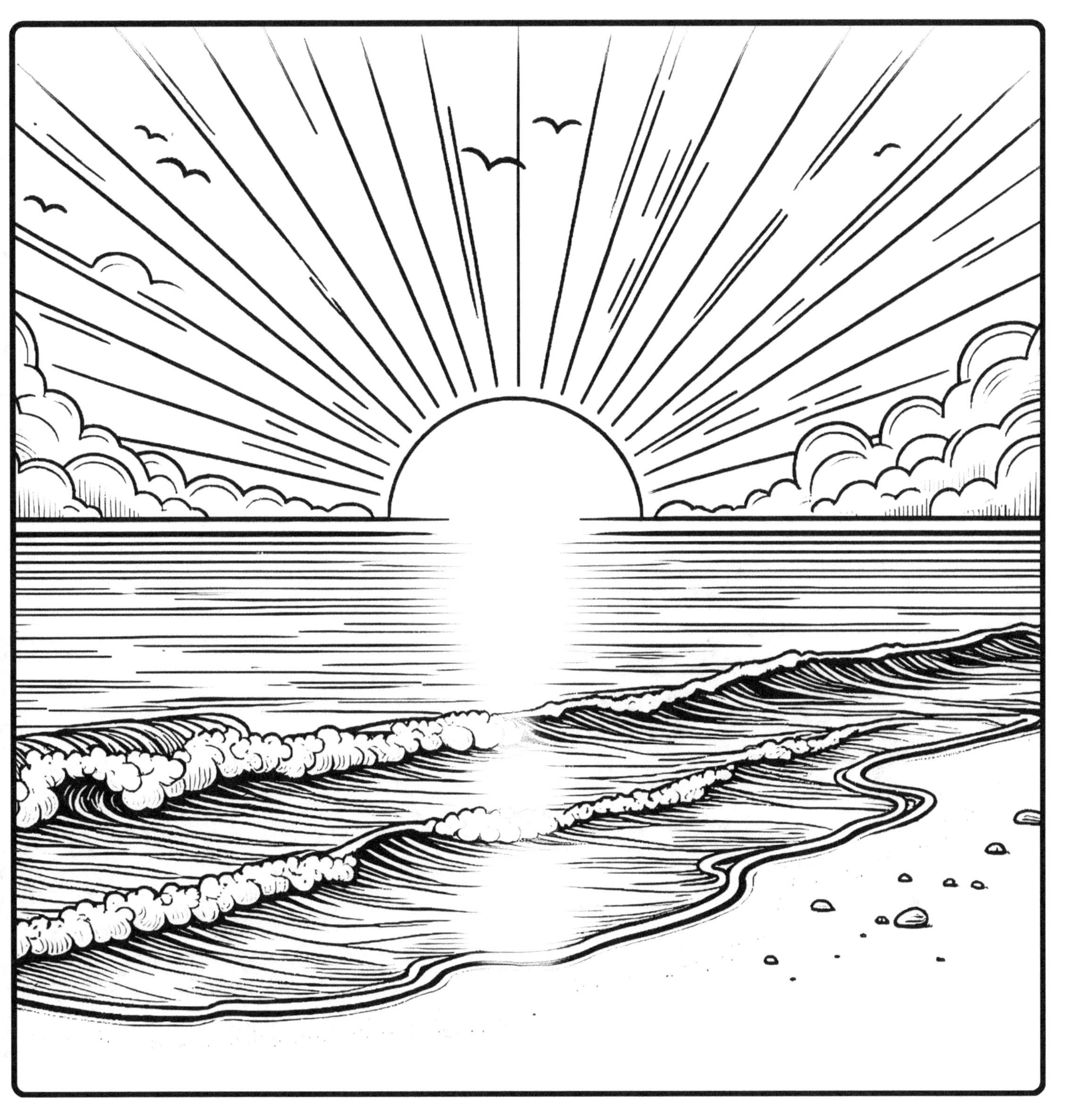

*"Breathe deeply and embrace
the joy of the moment."*

Growing Together

"Prepare a cozy space for your baby.
Creating a warm and loving environment will make them feel safe."

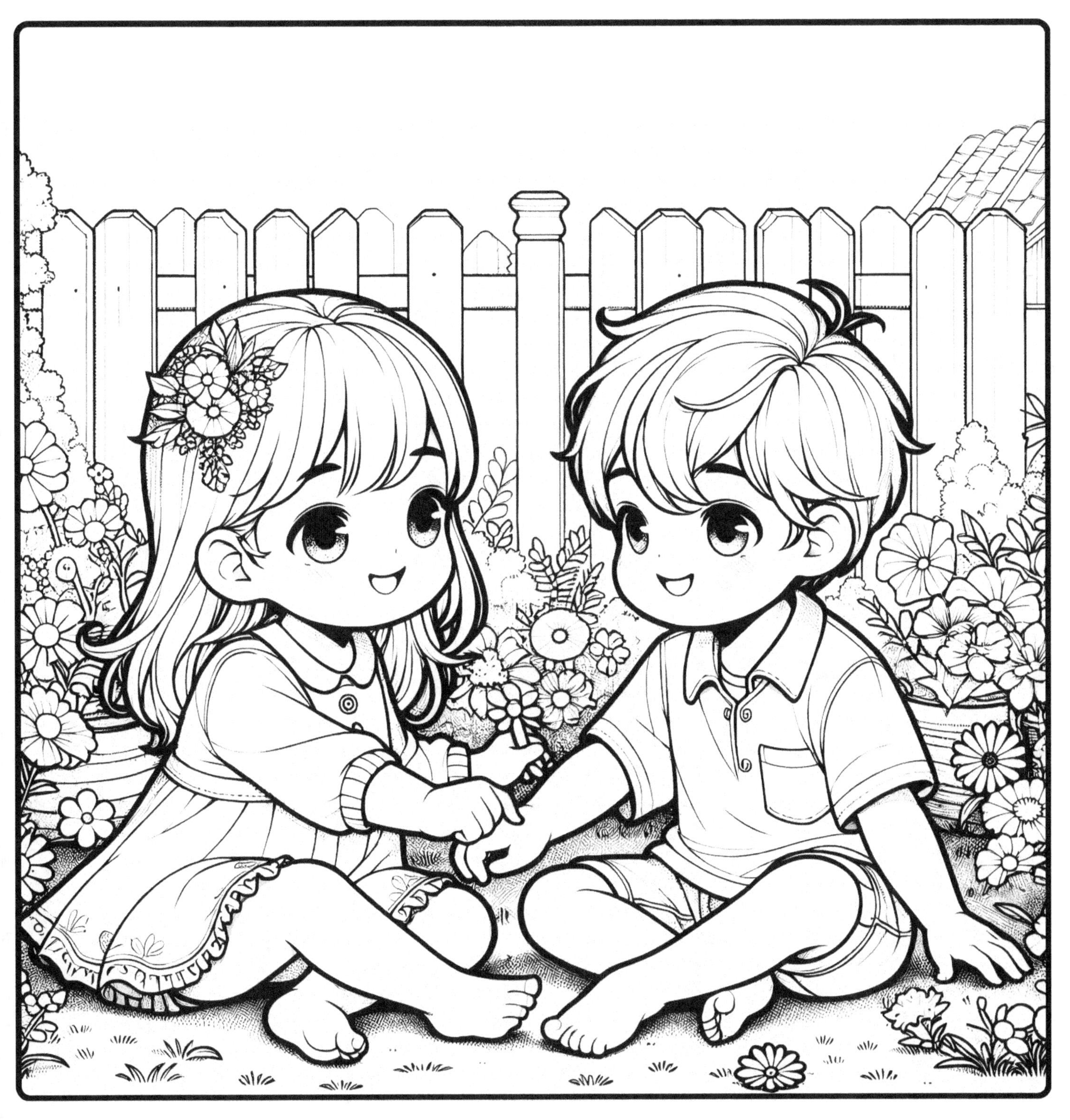

*"Joy is found
in the simplest moments."*

Growing Together

"Your baby's heart, brain, and spine are forming.
Isn't it amazing that your body is building a tiny human?"

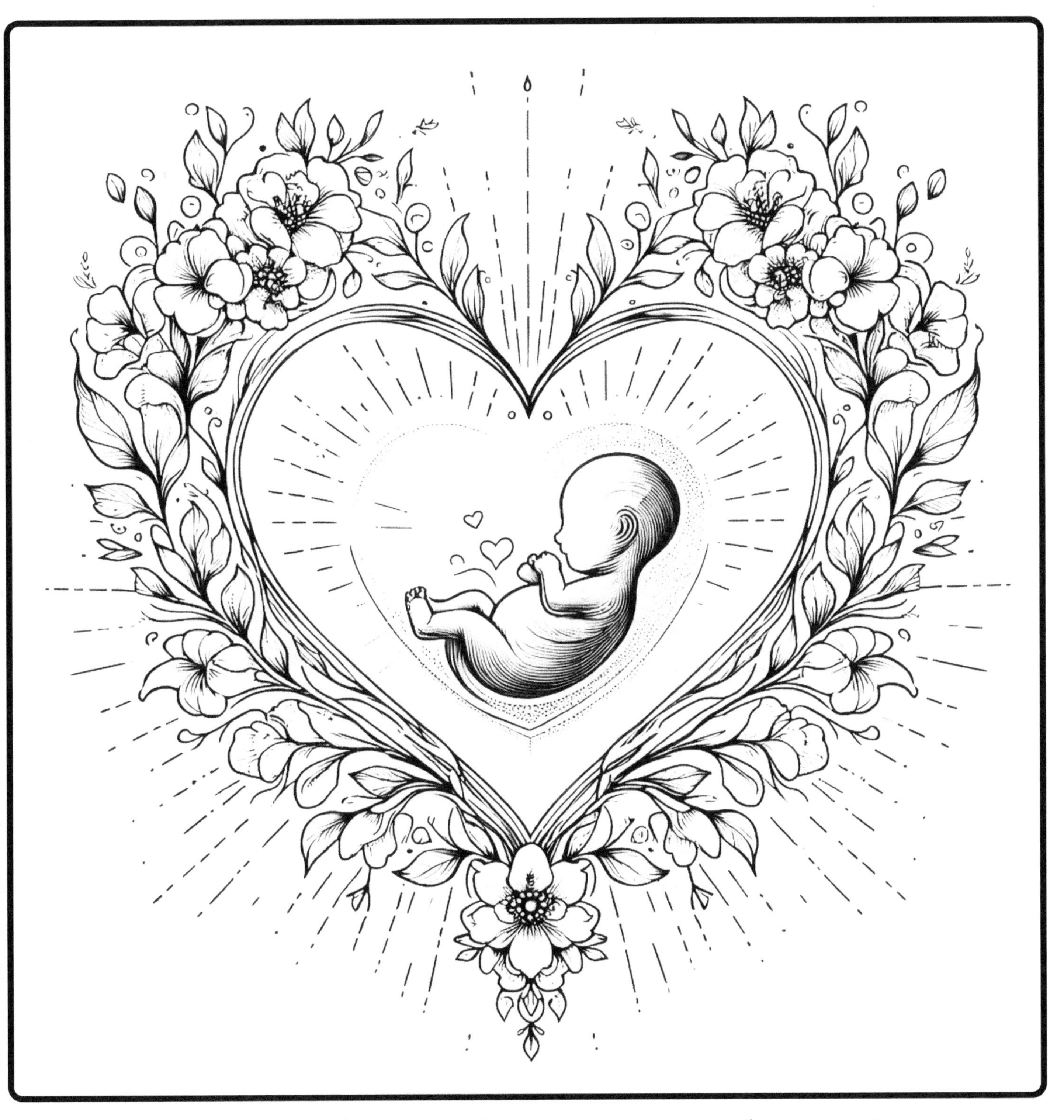

"Every heartbeat is a step closer
to meeting your little one."

Growing Together

"Do what makes you happy,
like listening to your favorite music or reading a good book.
Little joys matter!"

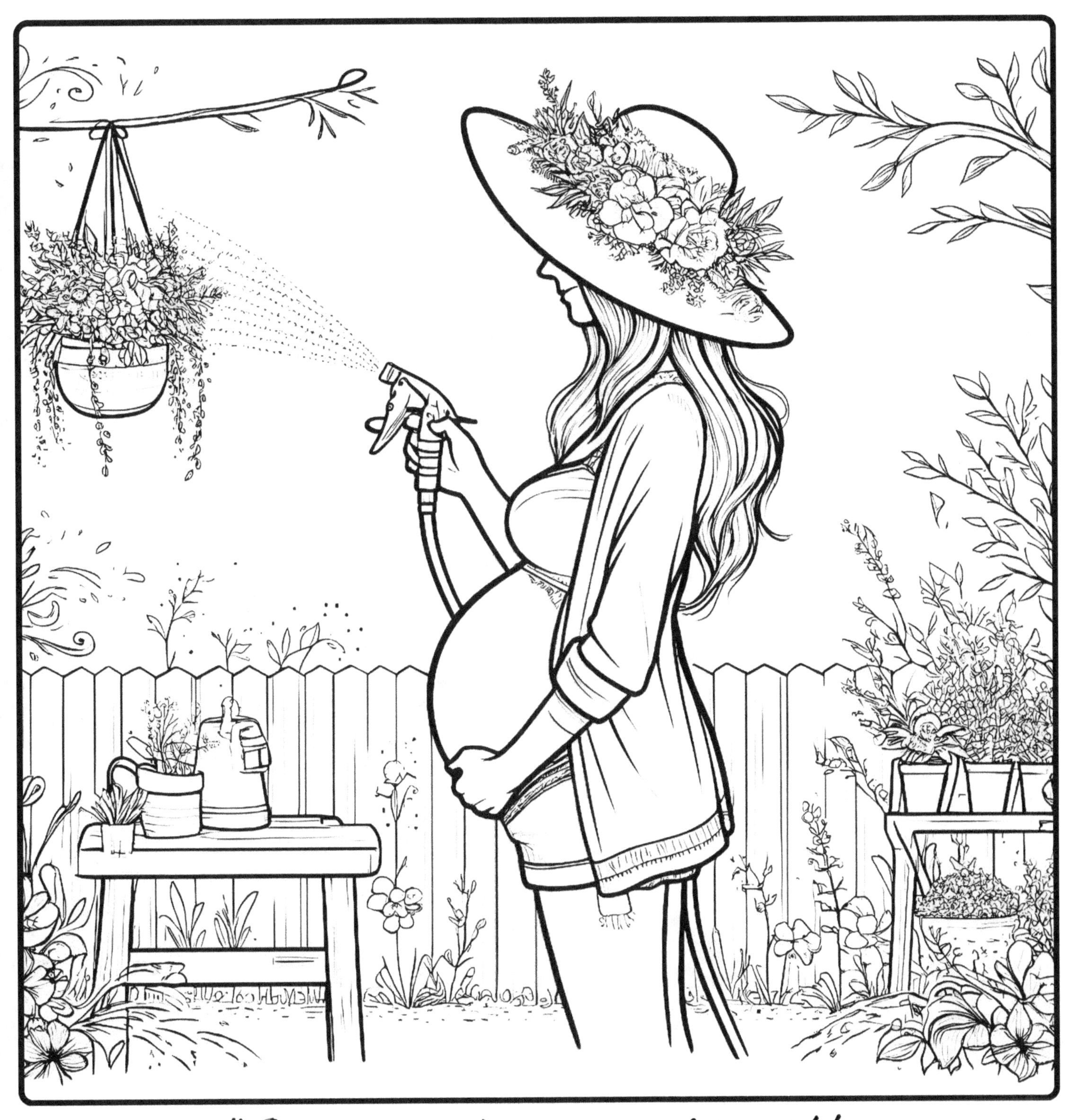

"Surround yourself with love and light."

Growing Together

"Trust your body, it knows what to do.
You're like a superhero with an amazing power."

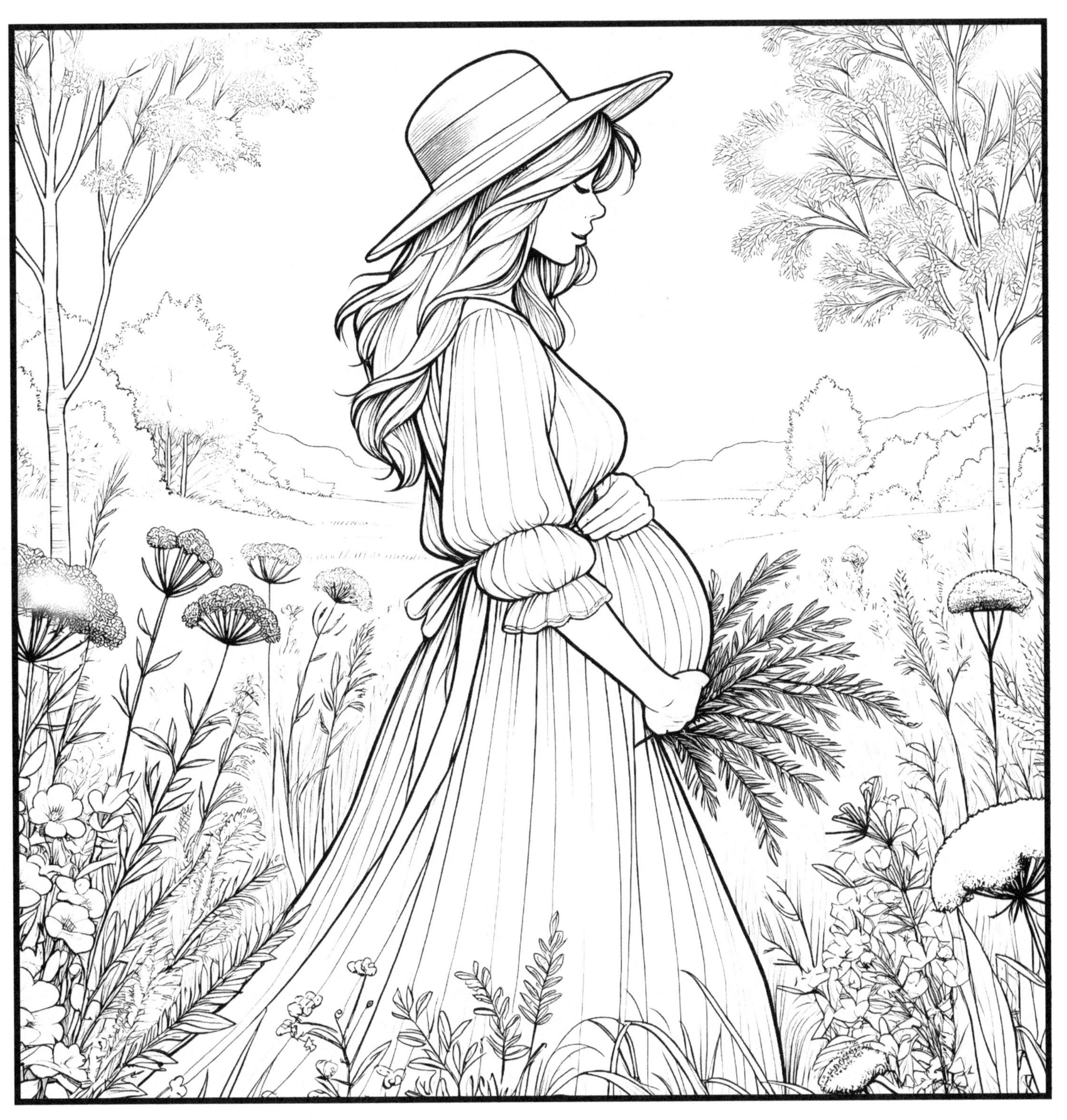

"Embrace the changes
and cherish the journey."

Growing Together

"You have an amazing ability to care for your baby.
Believe in your inner strength."

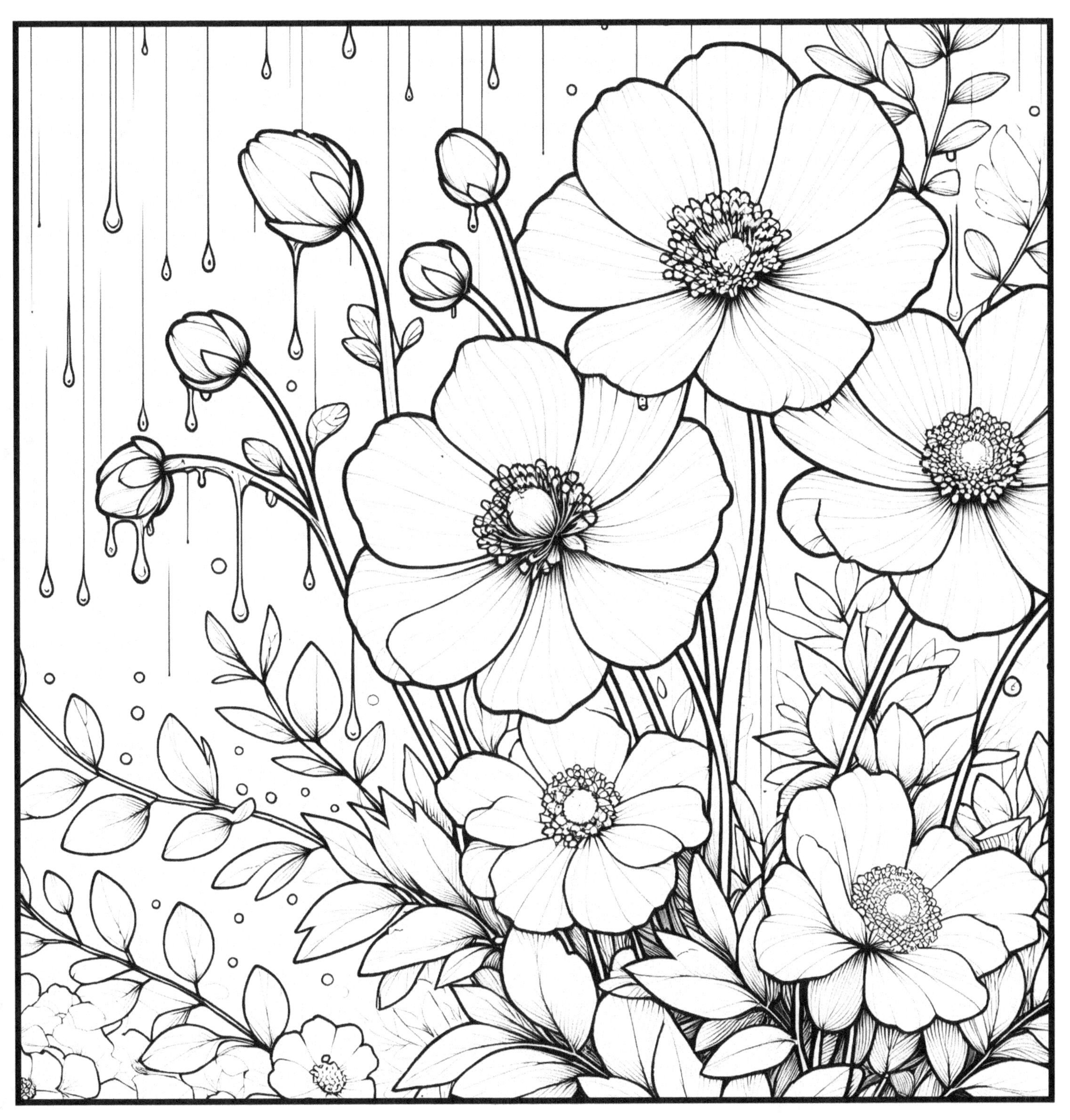

"You are a beautiful work
in progress."

Growing Together

"Doing activities that make you feel relaxed and happy,
like reading, watching movies, or crafting,
will reduce stress and increase happiness."

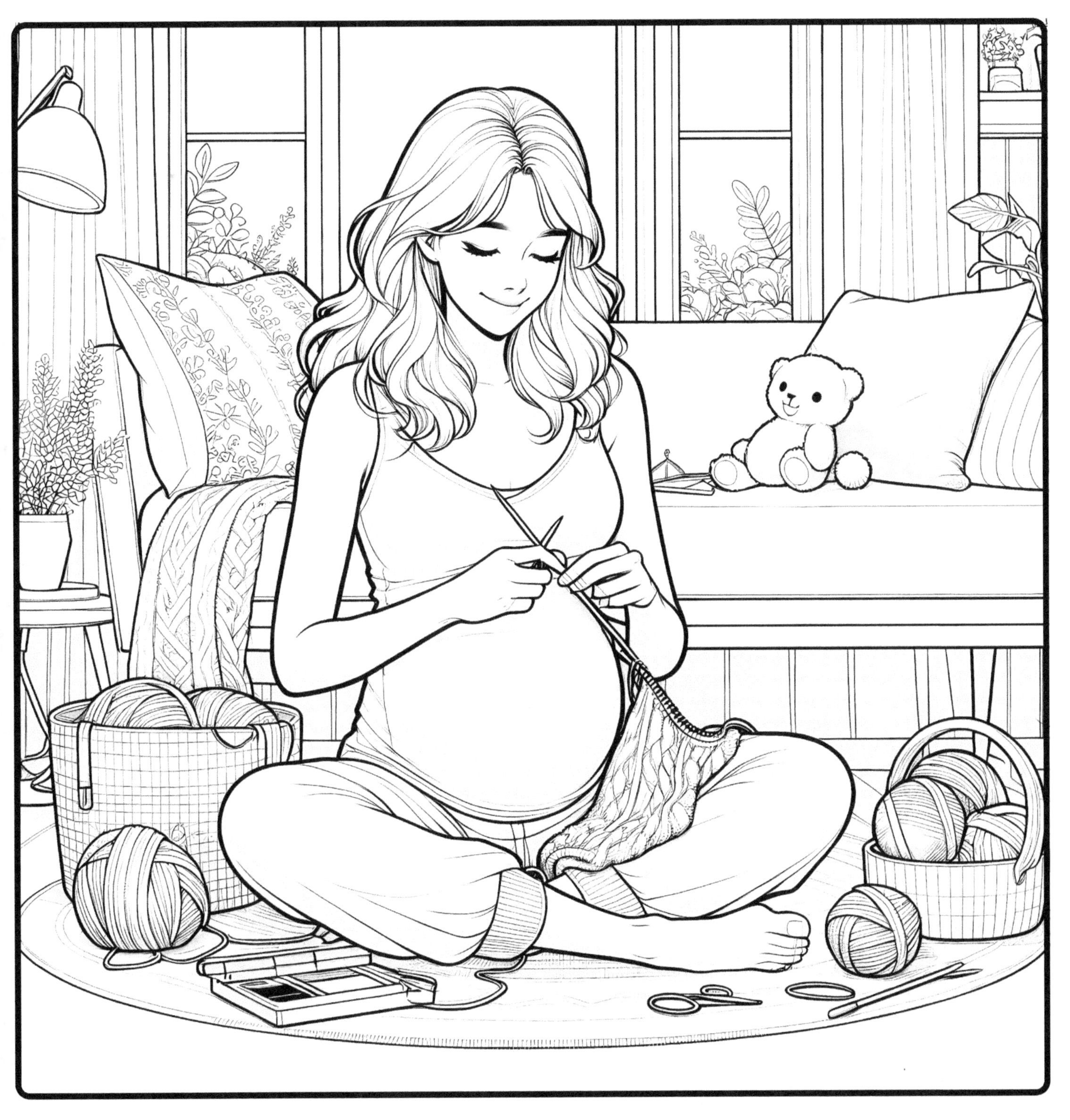

"The bond between you and
your baby grows stronger every day."

Growing
Together

"Feeling tired?
Take a nap!
Your body is doing a lot of hard work."

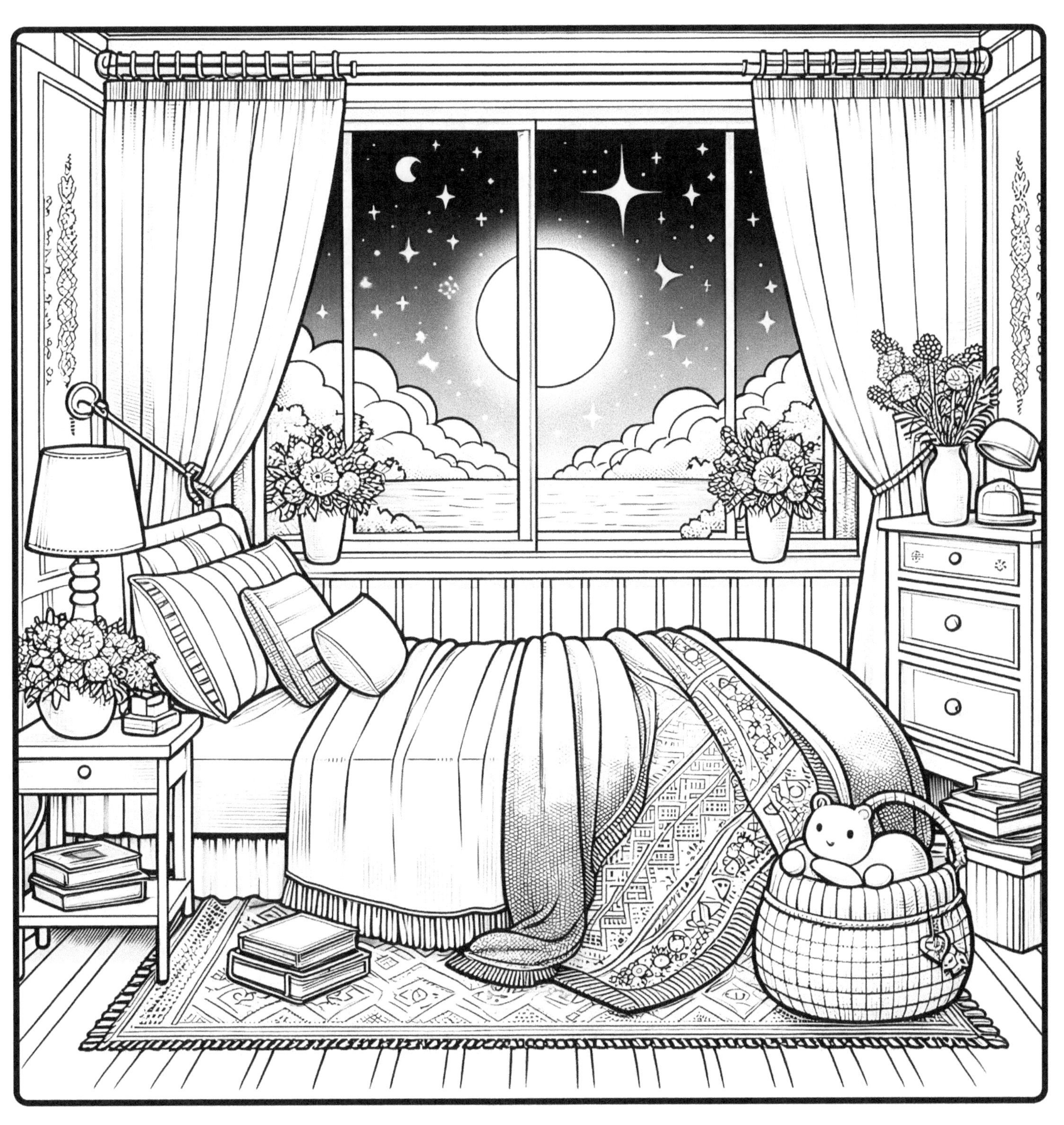

*"Take time to relax
and enjoy this special journey."*

Growing Together

"Take care of both your body and mind.
Meditate, listen to music, and relax."

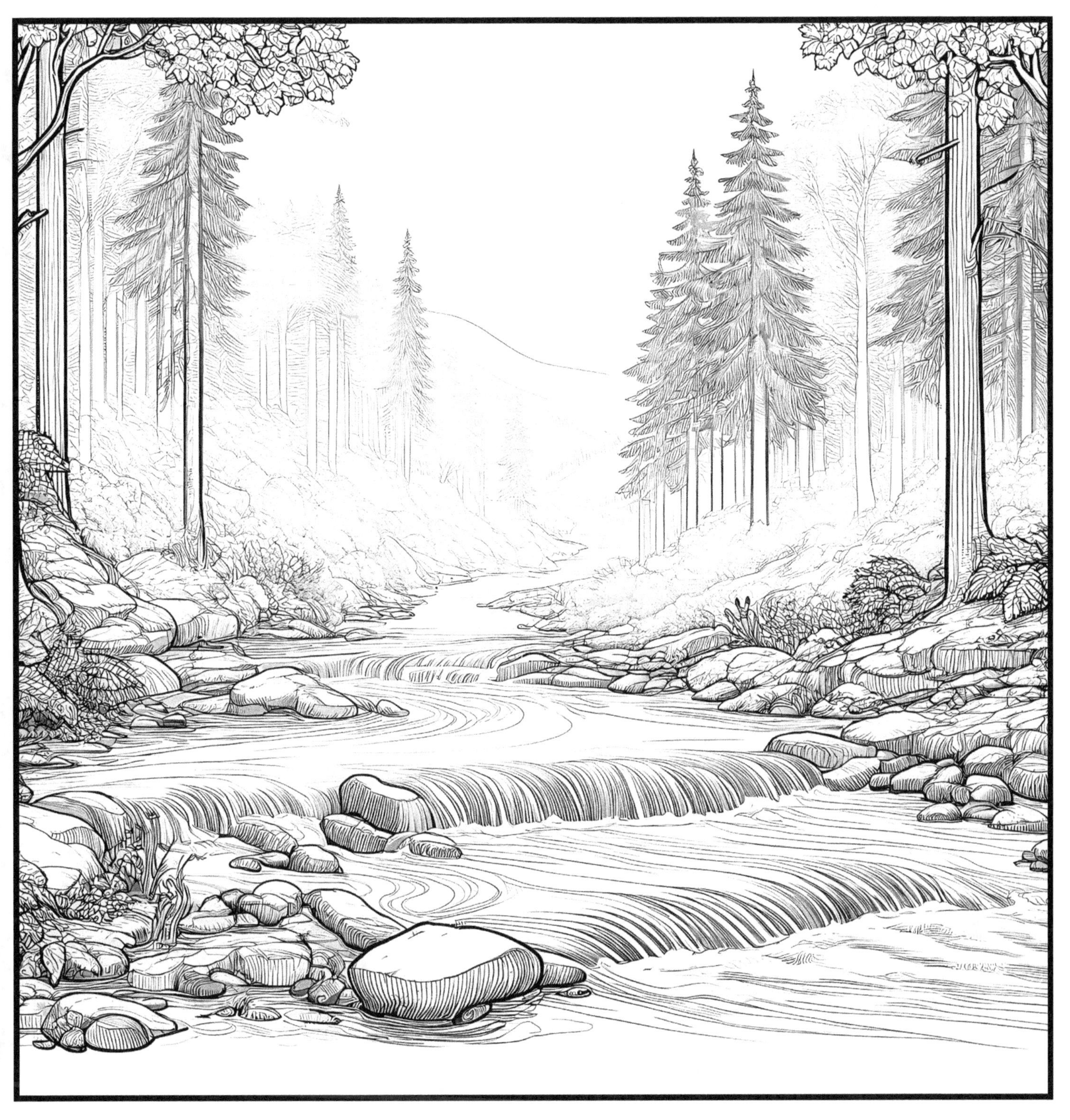

*"The love you have for your baby
is already immeasurable."*

Growing Together

"Celebrate every little kick and flutter.
These moments are precious."

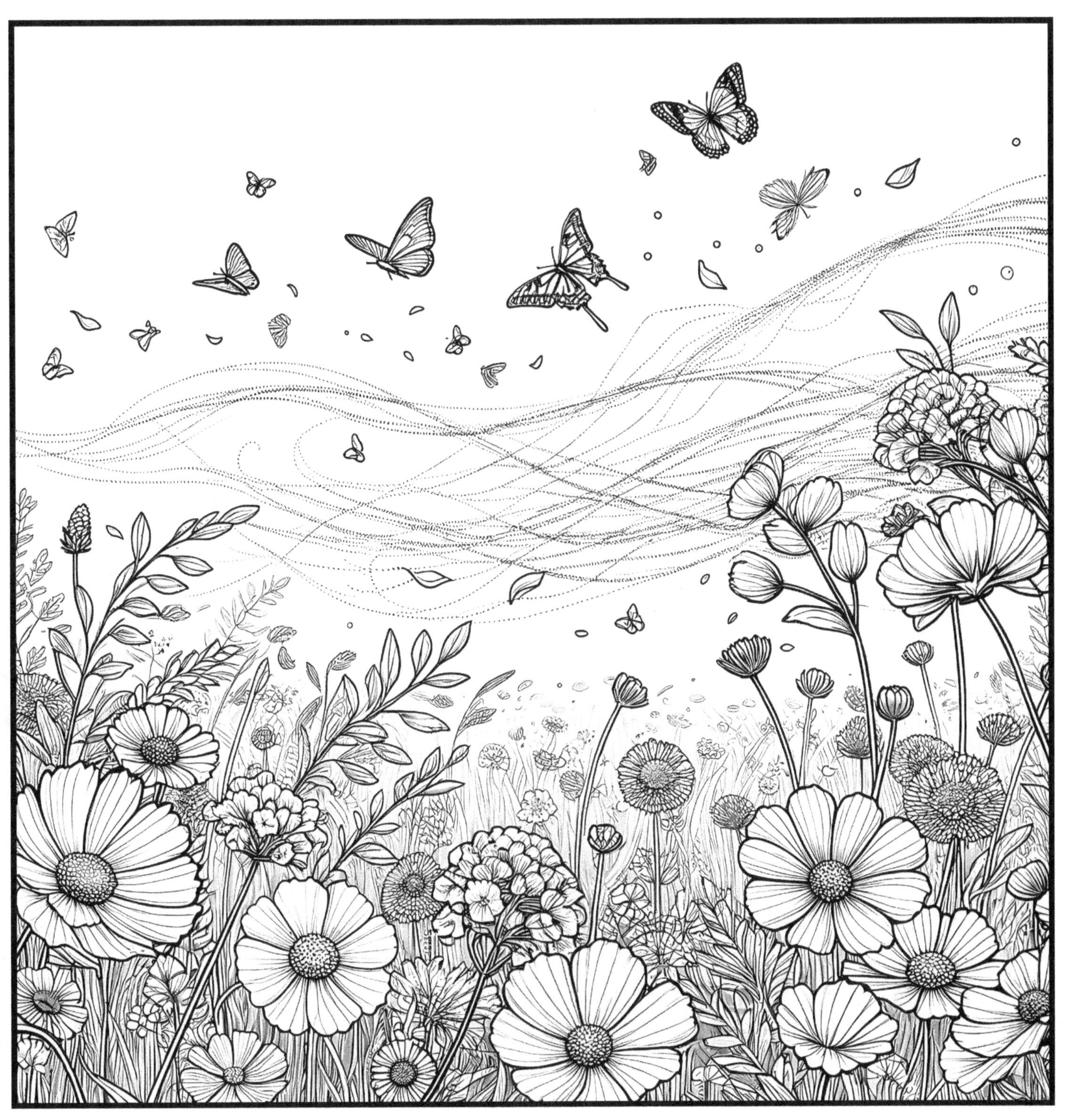

"Cherish the little kicks
and flutters."

Growing
Together

"Pregnancy is a journey filled with hope and happiness.
Enjoy every step with love."

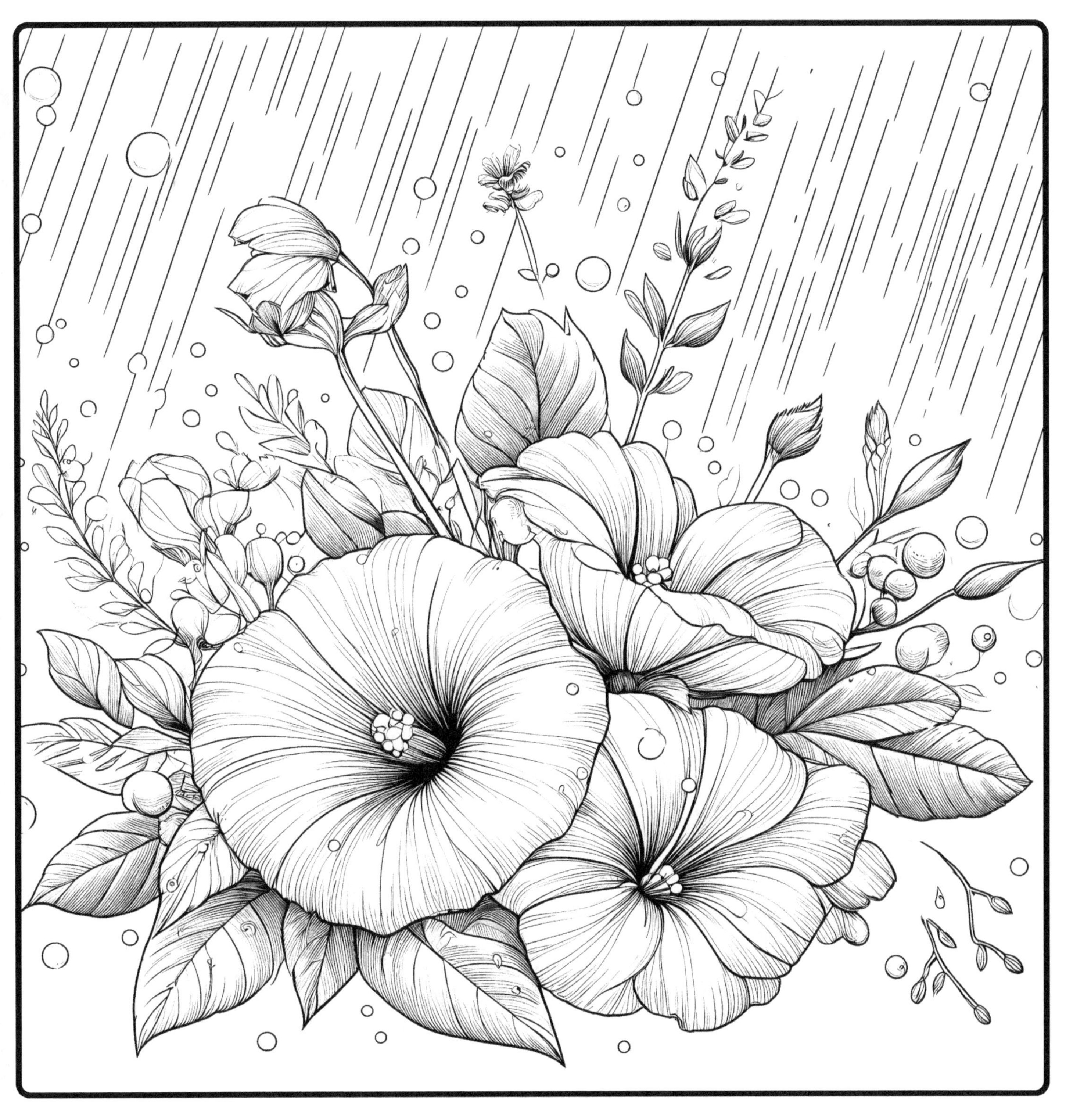

"You are strong,
beautiful, and capable."

Growing
Together

"Your baby is growing with your love.
Keep nurturing them with your heart."

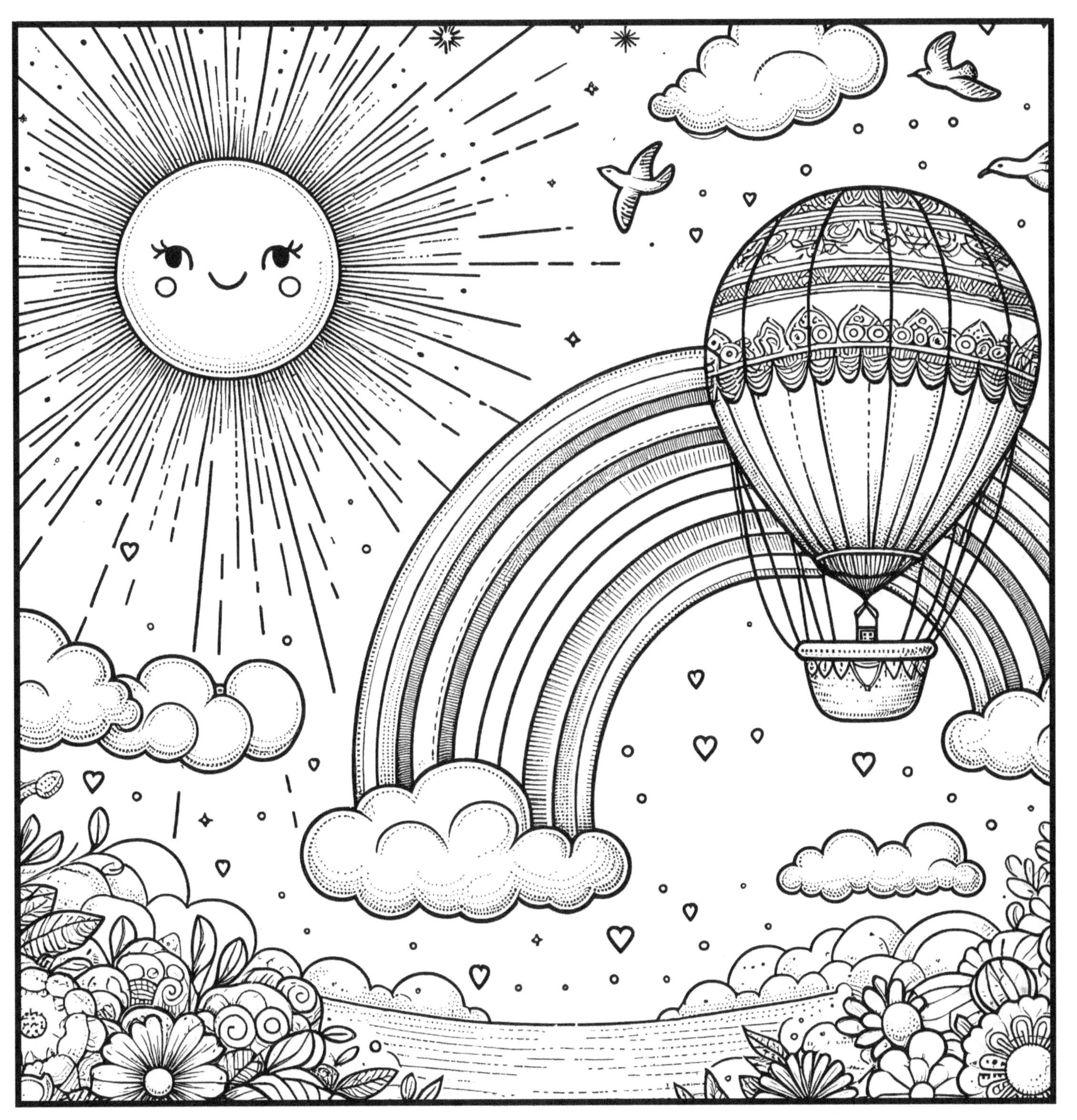

"Each day brings new joys
and wonders."

Growing Together

"Your love and care are already shaping your baby's future.
Trust in your ability to nurture and protect them."

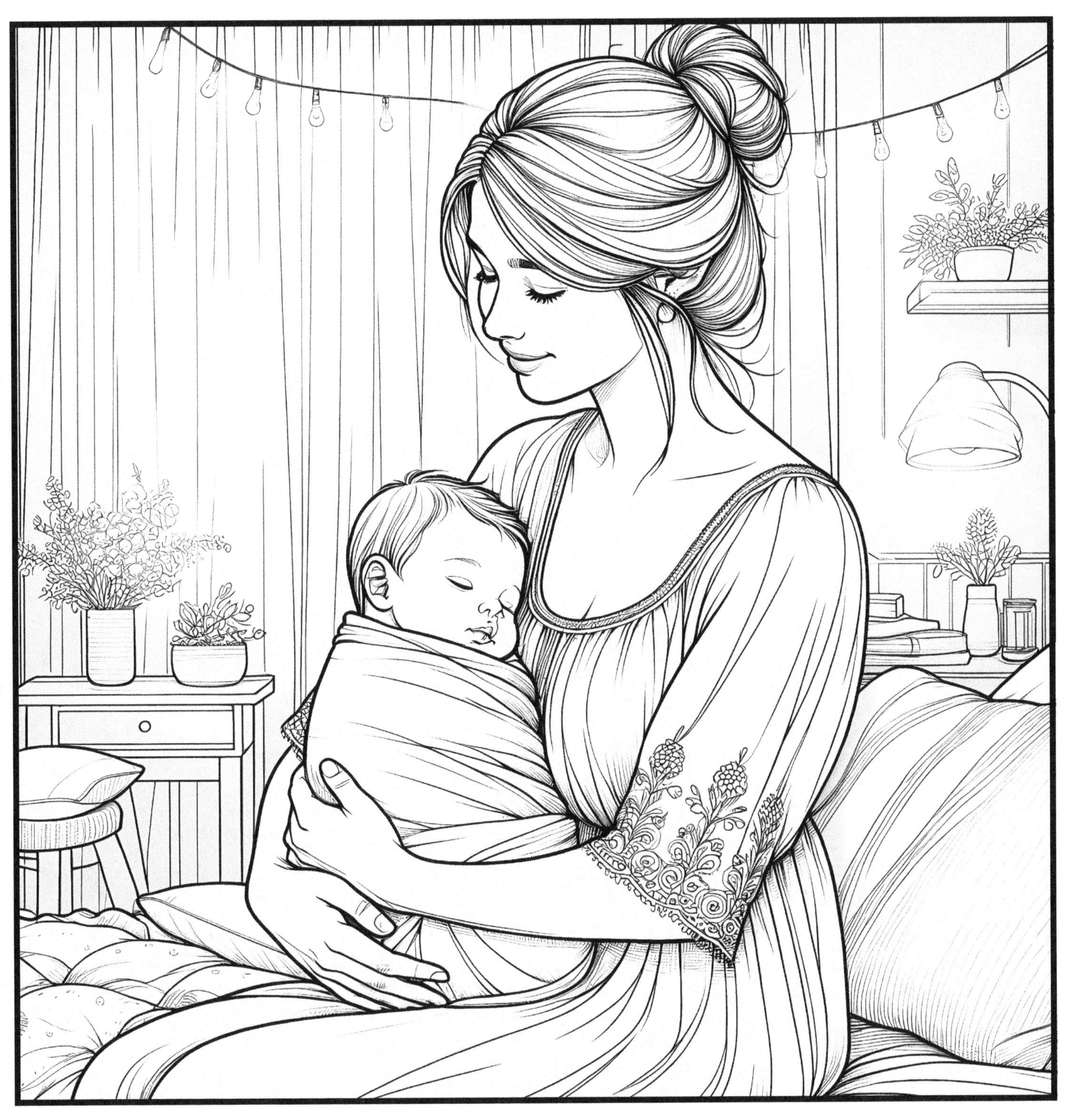

*"Embrace the journey
with an open heart."*

Growing Together

"Eating nutritious foods helps your baby grow strong.
Think of it as feeding a tiny superhero!"

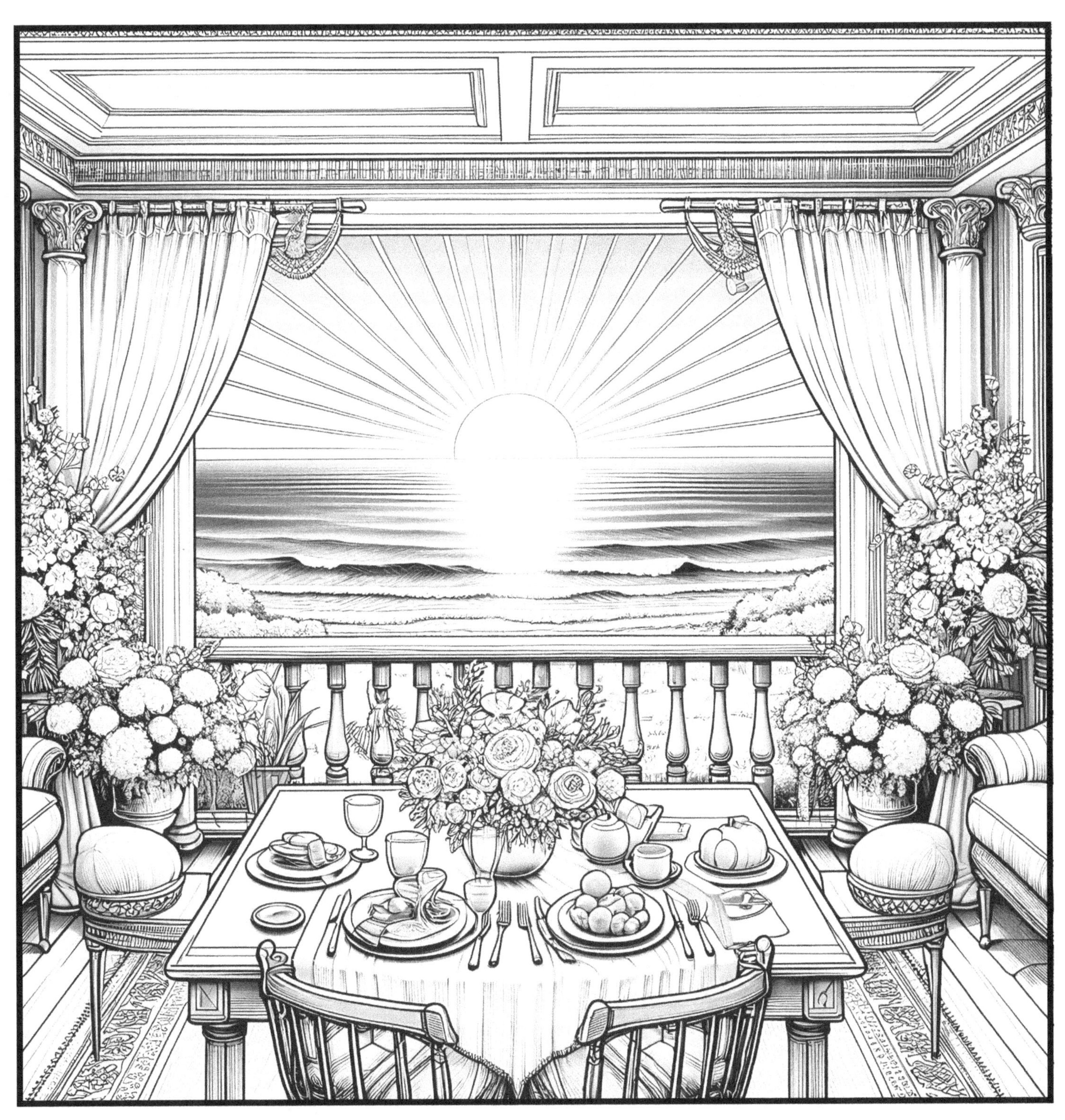

"Your love is the foundation
of a new life."

Growing
Together

"The love you have for your baby is limitless.
It gives you incredible strength."

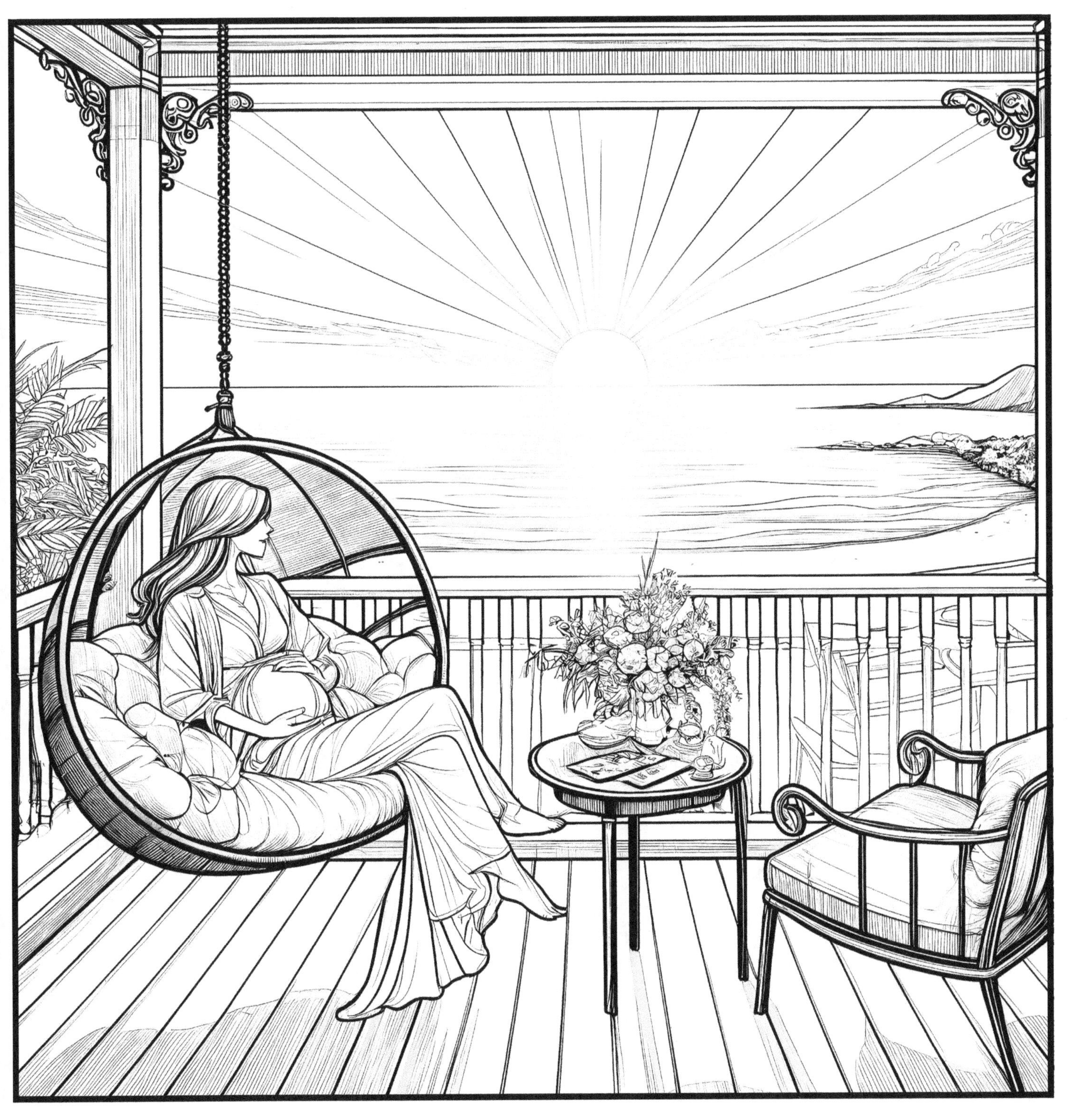

*"Breathe, relax,
and enjoy each moment."*

Growing Together

"Practice deep breathing and enjoy the calm it brings.
You deserve all the peace."

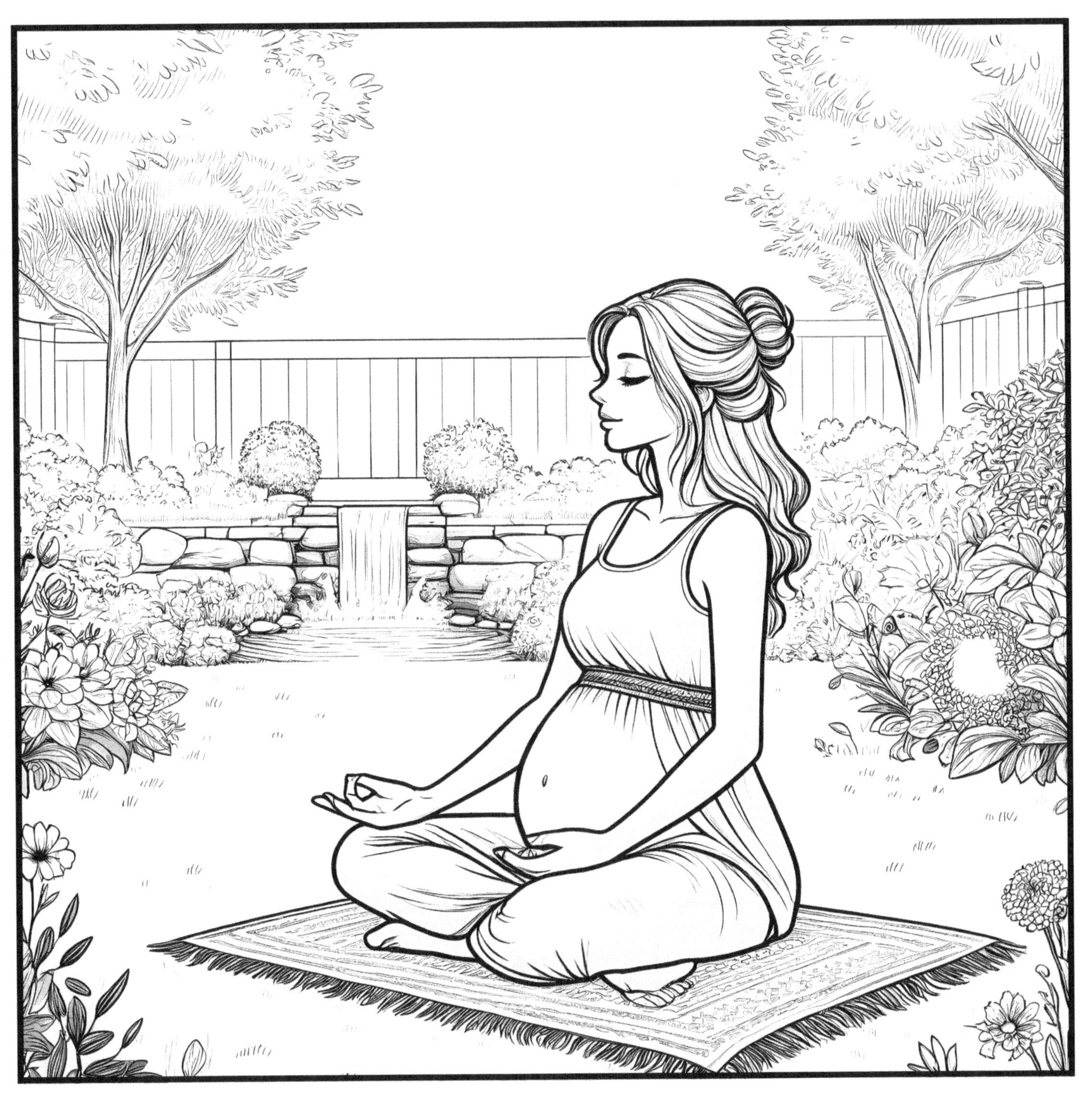

"Your body is amazing
and powerful."

Growing Together

"Rest and relax whenever you can.
Picture yourself as a serene, glowing goddess."

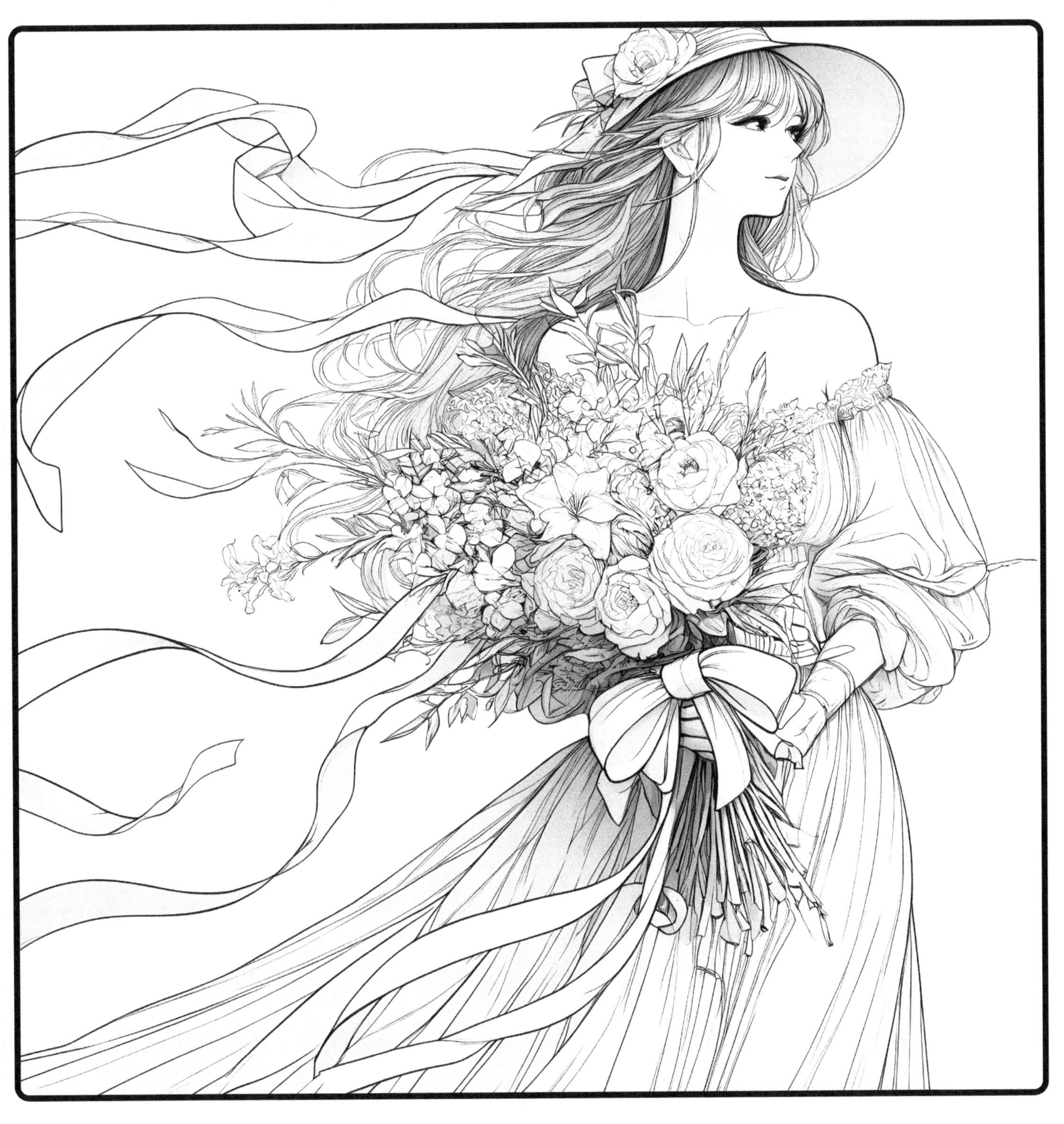

"Celebrate the miracle of life
growing within you."

Growing Together

"Every heartbeat you feel is a reminder of the new life growing inside you.
Cherish these precious moments."

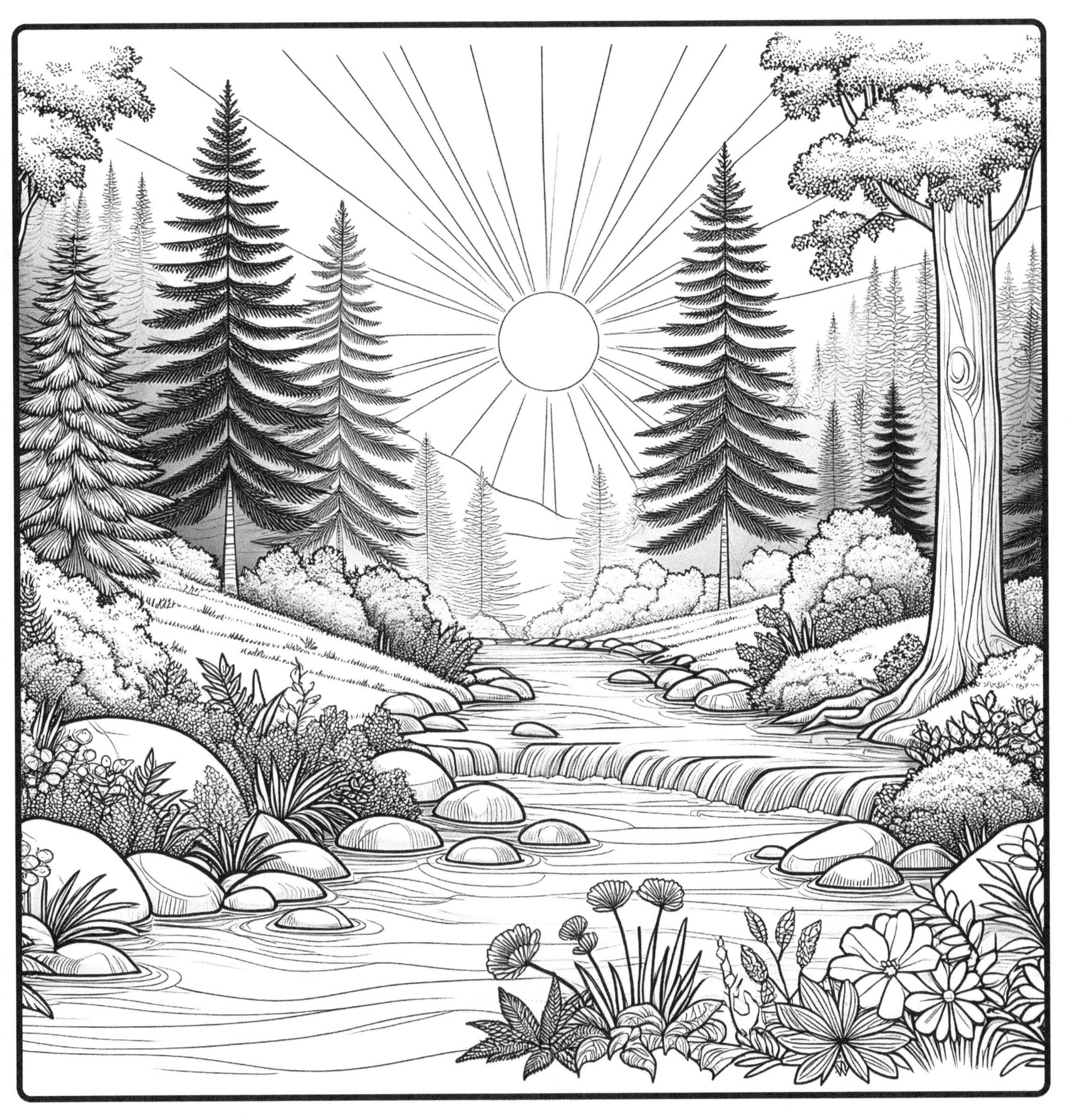

"You are surrounded by love and support."

Growing Together

"Taking care of yourself is taking care of your baby.
Prioritize rest, nutrition, and happiness."

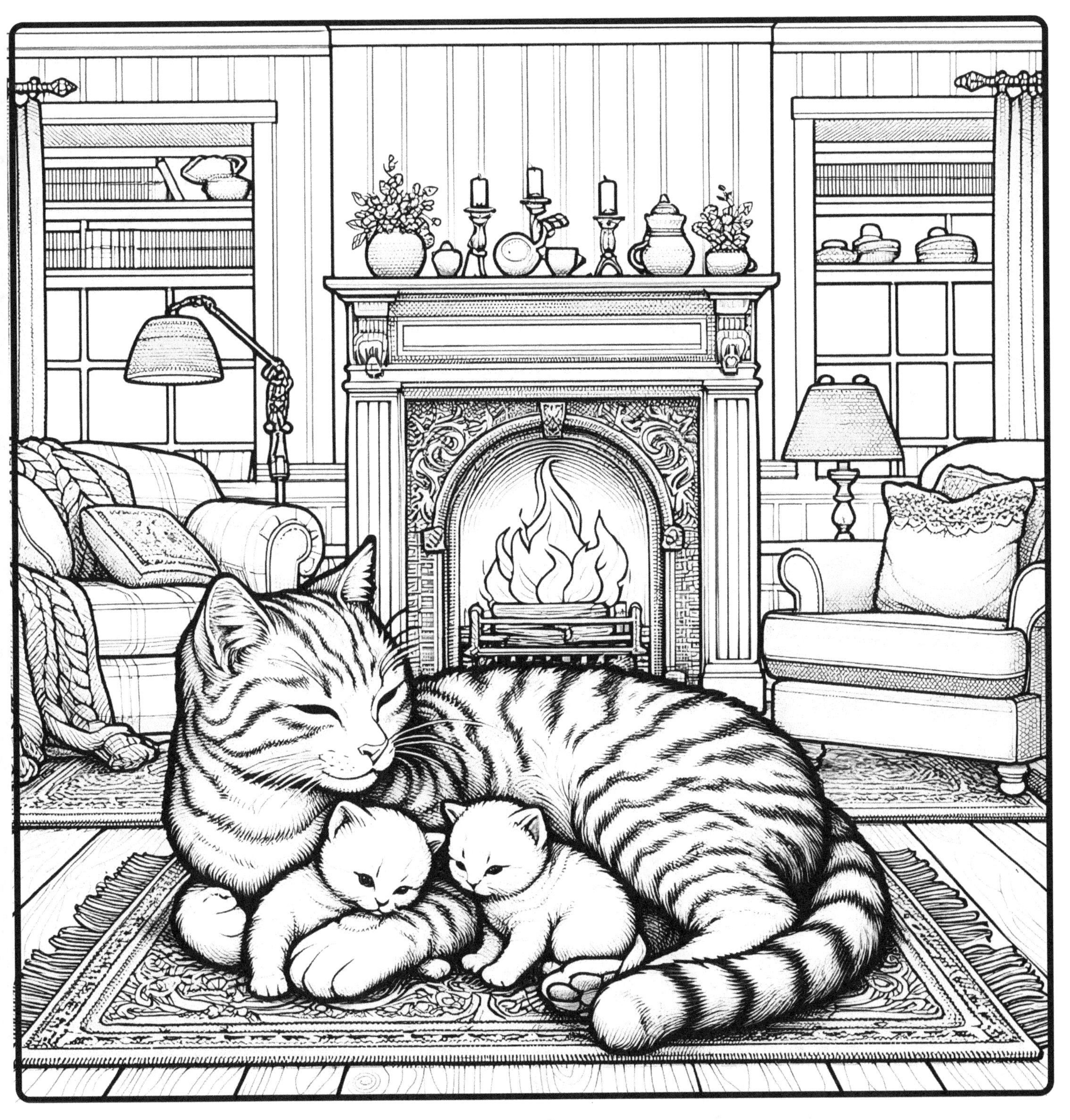

"Every moment is a precious step in your journey."

Growing Together

"Talking to your baby can create a special bond.
Go ahead, tell them about your day!"

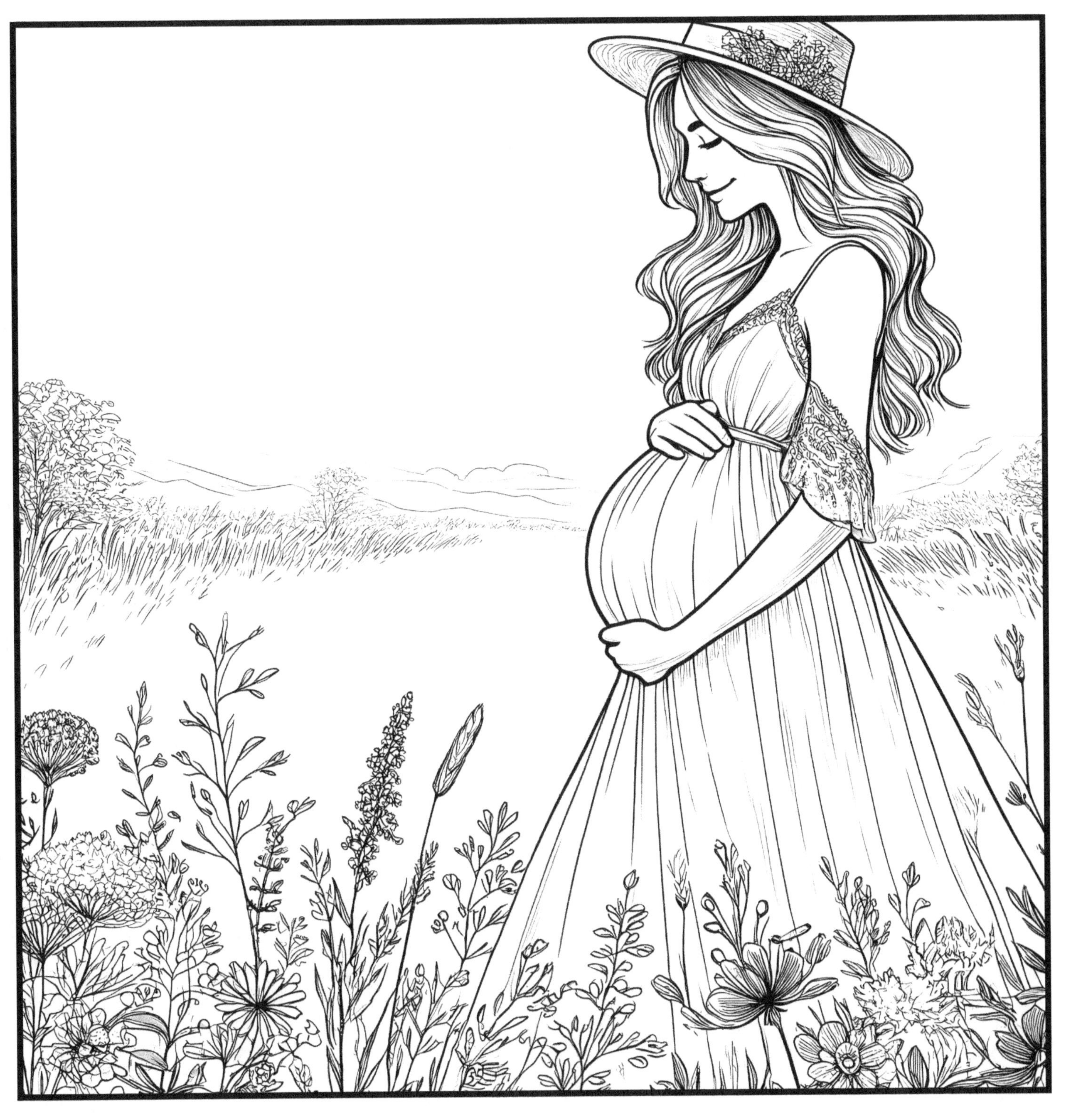

*"Nurture yourself
as you nurture your baby."*

Growing Together

"Your body is doing something extraordinary.
Appreciate its strength and beauty during this time."

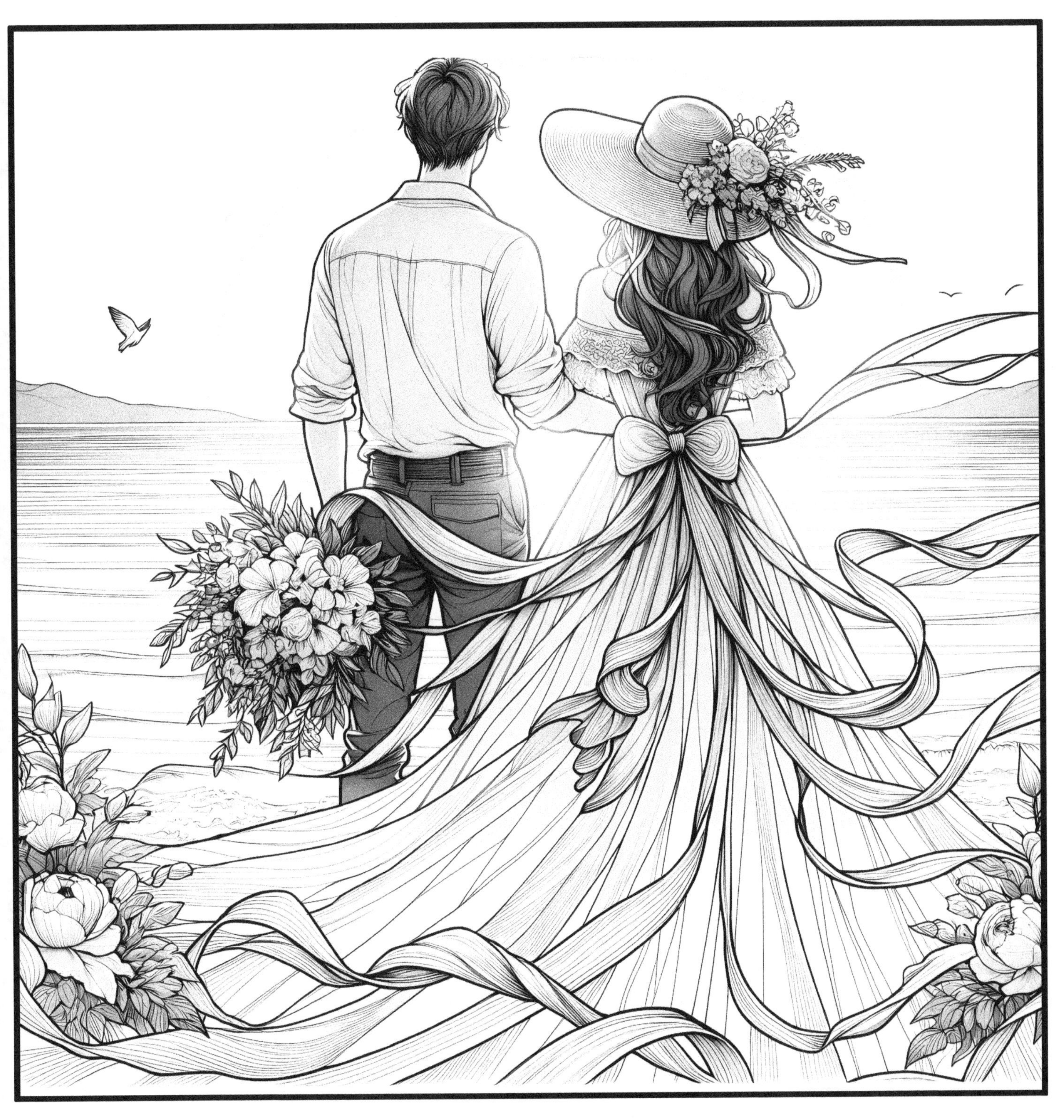

The best is yet to come.

Growing Together

"Embrace the changes your body is going through.
Each change is a sign of the amazing work your body is doing."

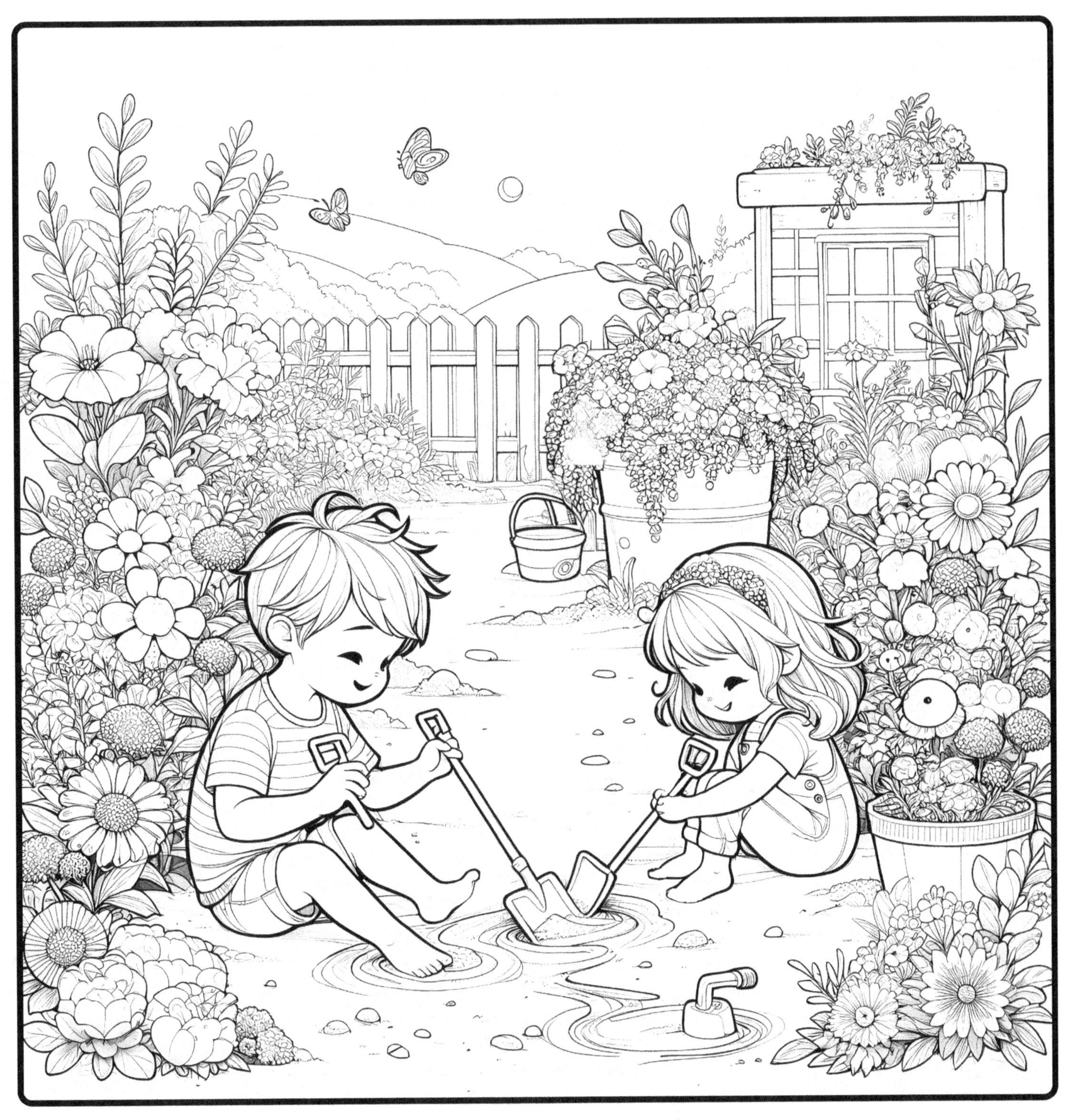

"You are creating
a beautiful life."

Growing Together

"Joy is found in the little things.
Your smile is a gift to the world!"

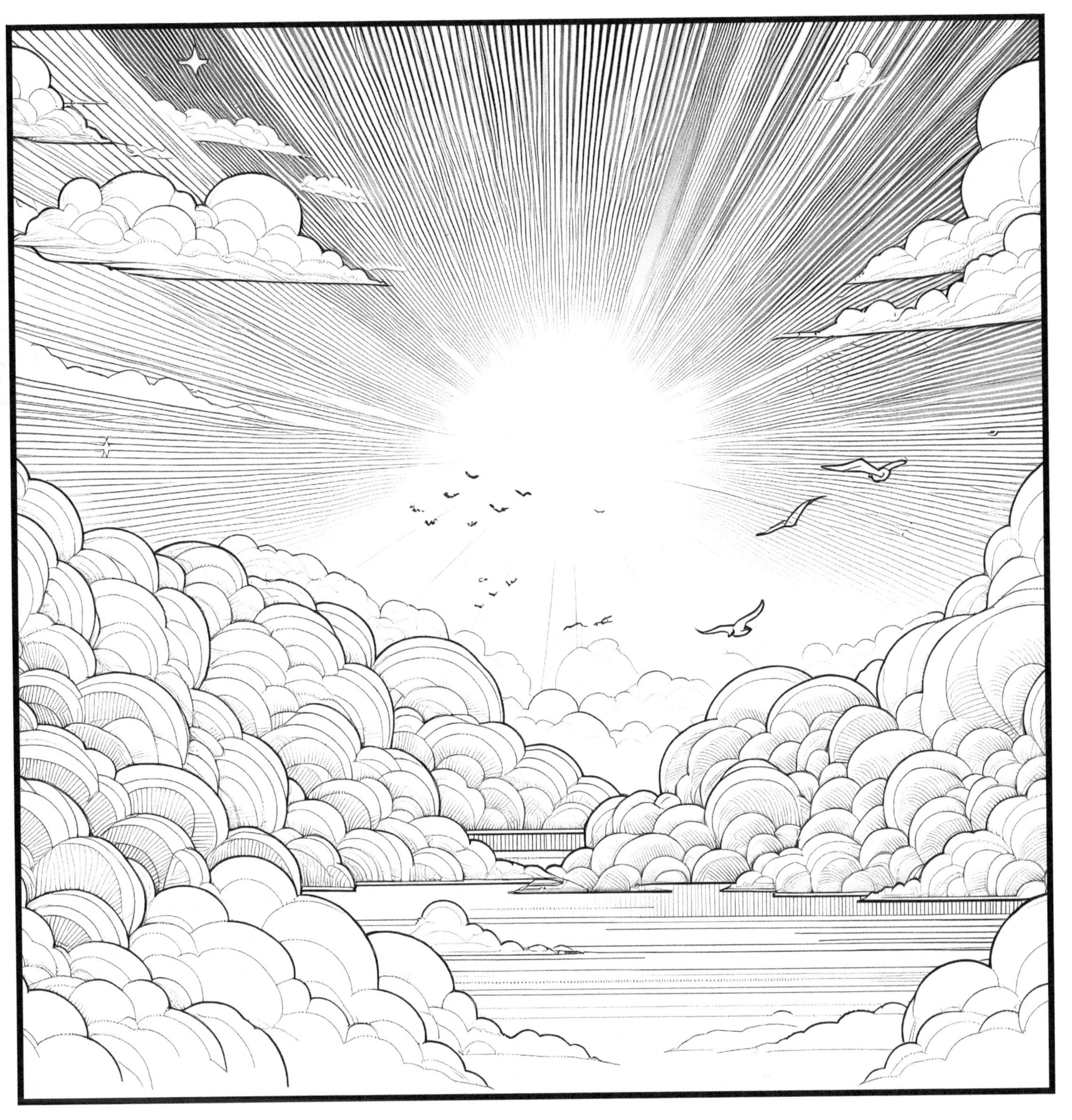

"Your journey is unique
and wonderful."

Growing
Together

"Enjoy the journey and take it one day at a time.
Every day brings you closer to meeting your little one."

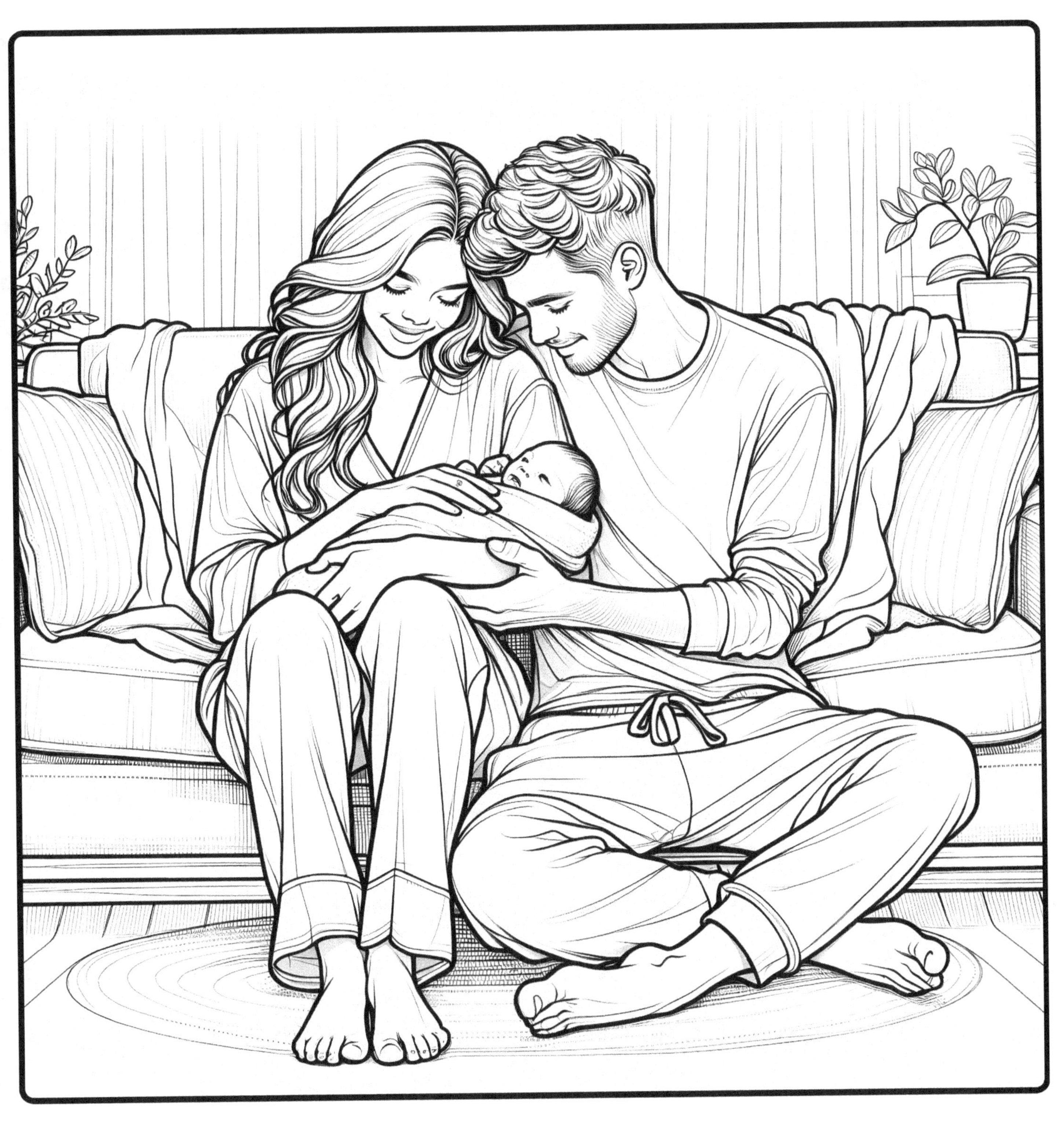

"Every day is a step closer to holding your baby."

Growing
Together

"Take time to relax and enjoy the little things.
Watch a funny movie or read a book you love."

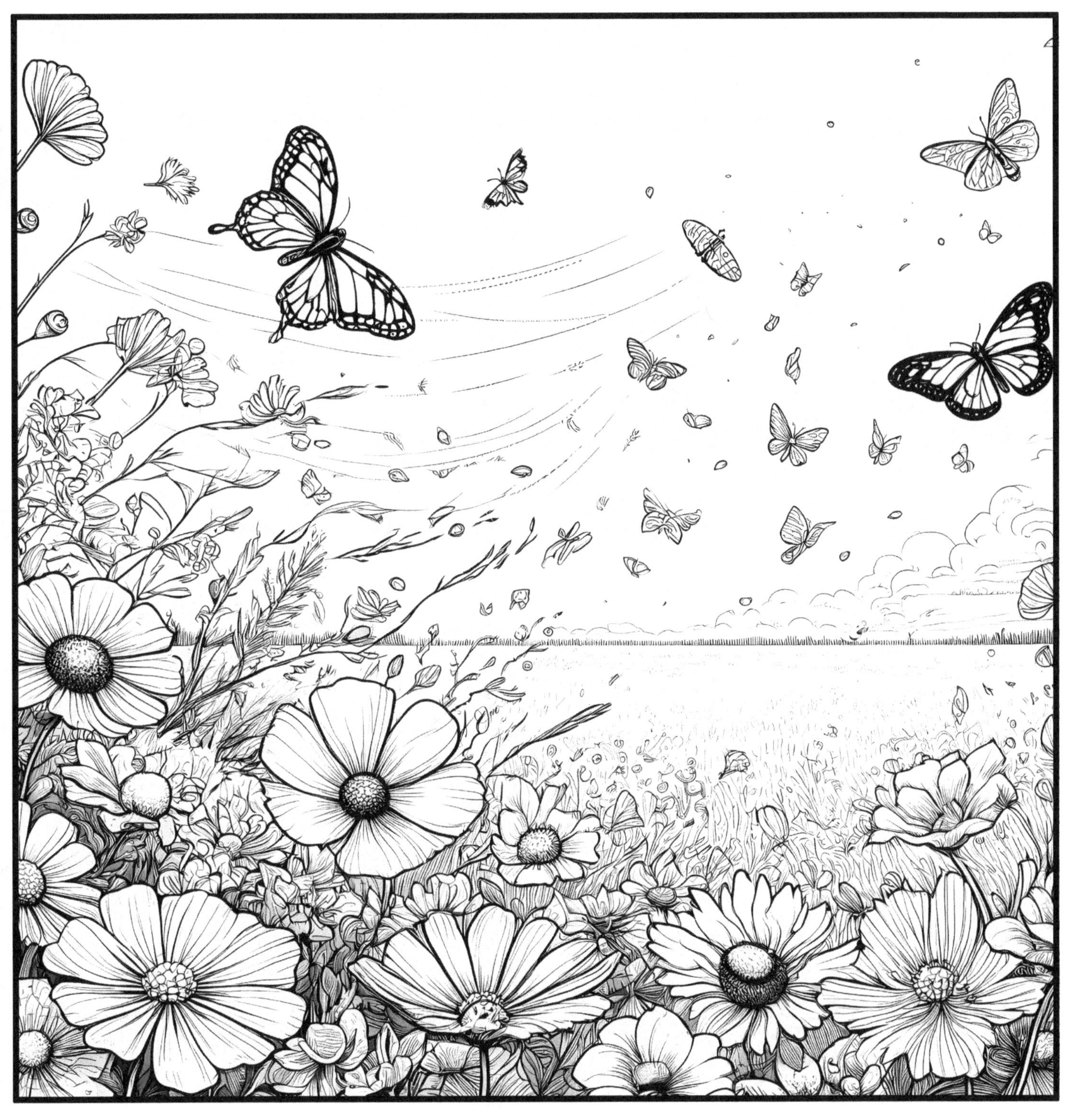

"The love you have
for your baby is boundless."

Growing Together

"Spend time with family and loved ones.
Their support is a precious gift."

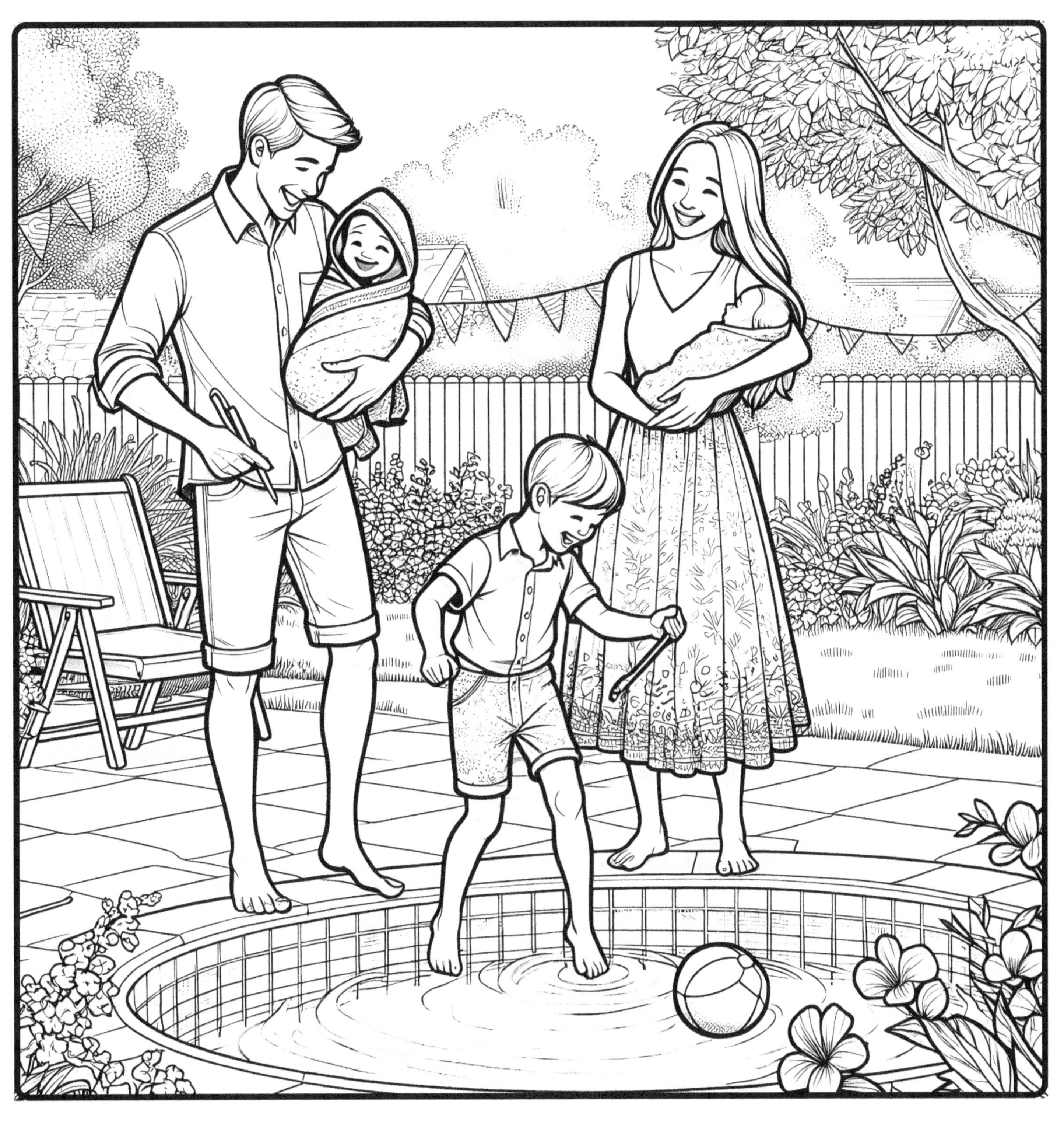

"Enjoy each moment
of this precious journey."

Growing Together

"Remember to stay hydrated.
Drinking enough water is essential for both you and your baby."

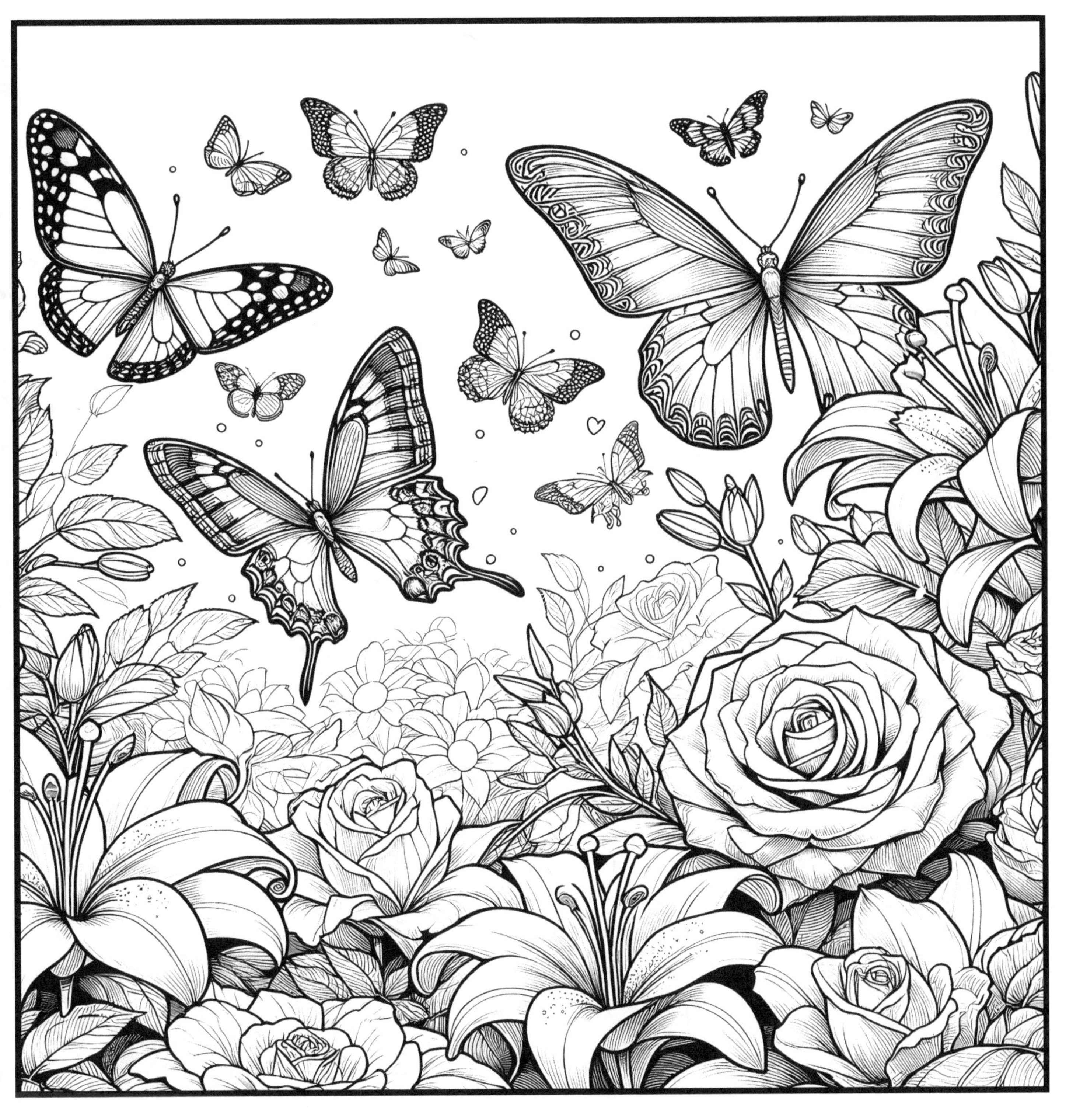

"You are a source of
life and love."

Growing Together

"You are creating a bond with your baby that will last a lifetime.
Talk to your baby and let them hear your voice."

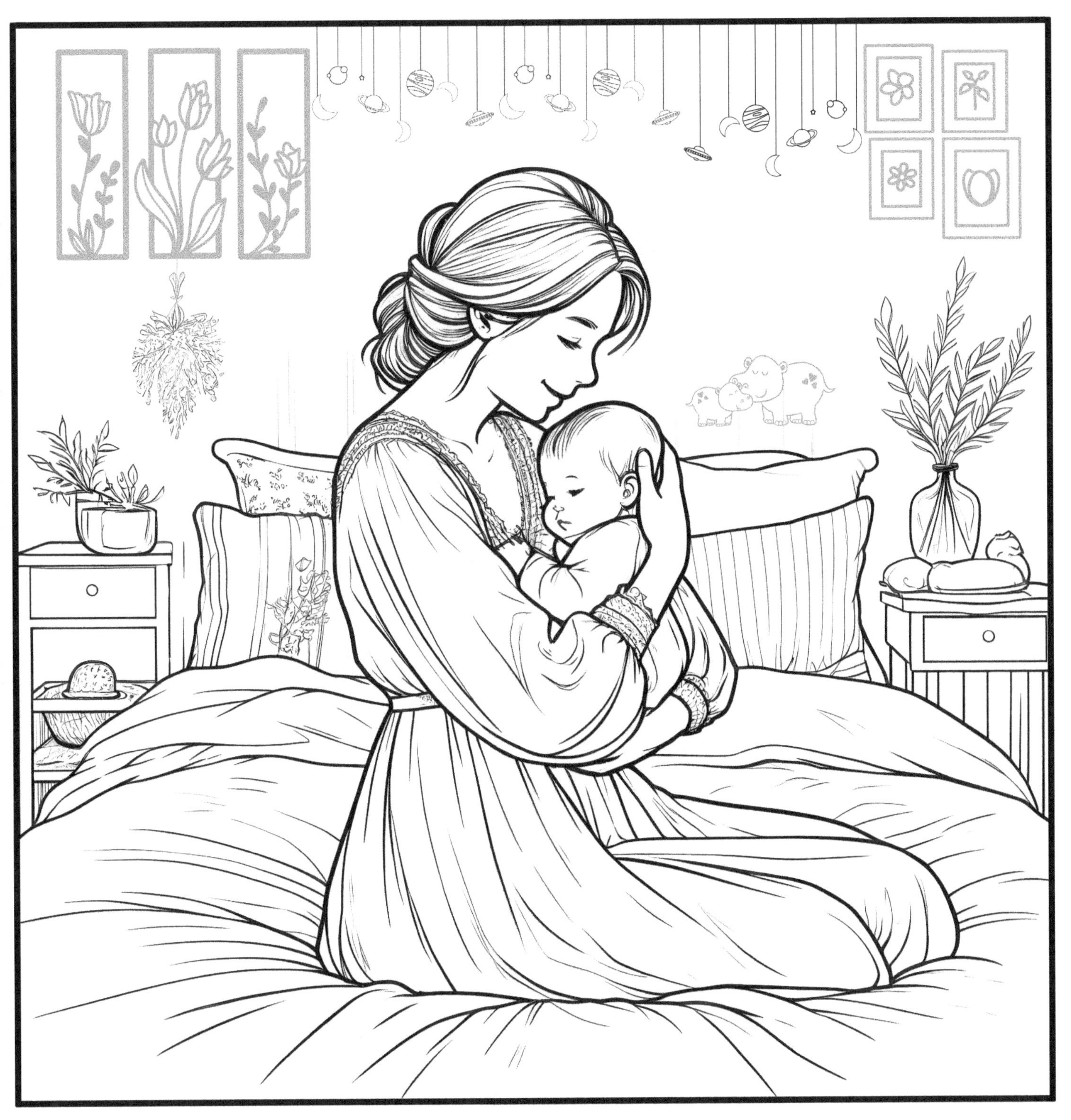

"You are strong, you are beautiful, you are a mother."

Growing Together

"Take care of your skin and pamper yourself.
You're glowing more every day!"

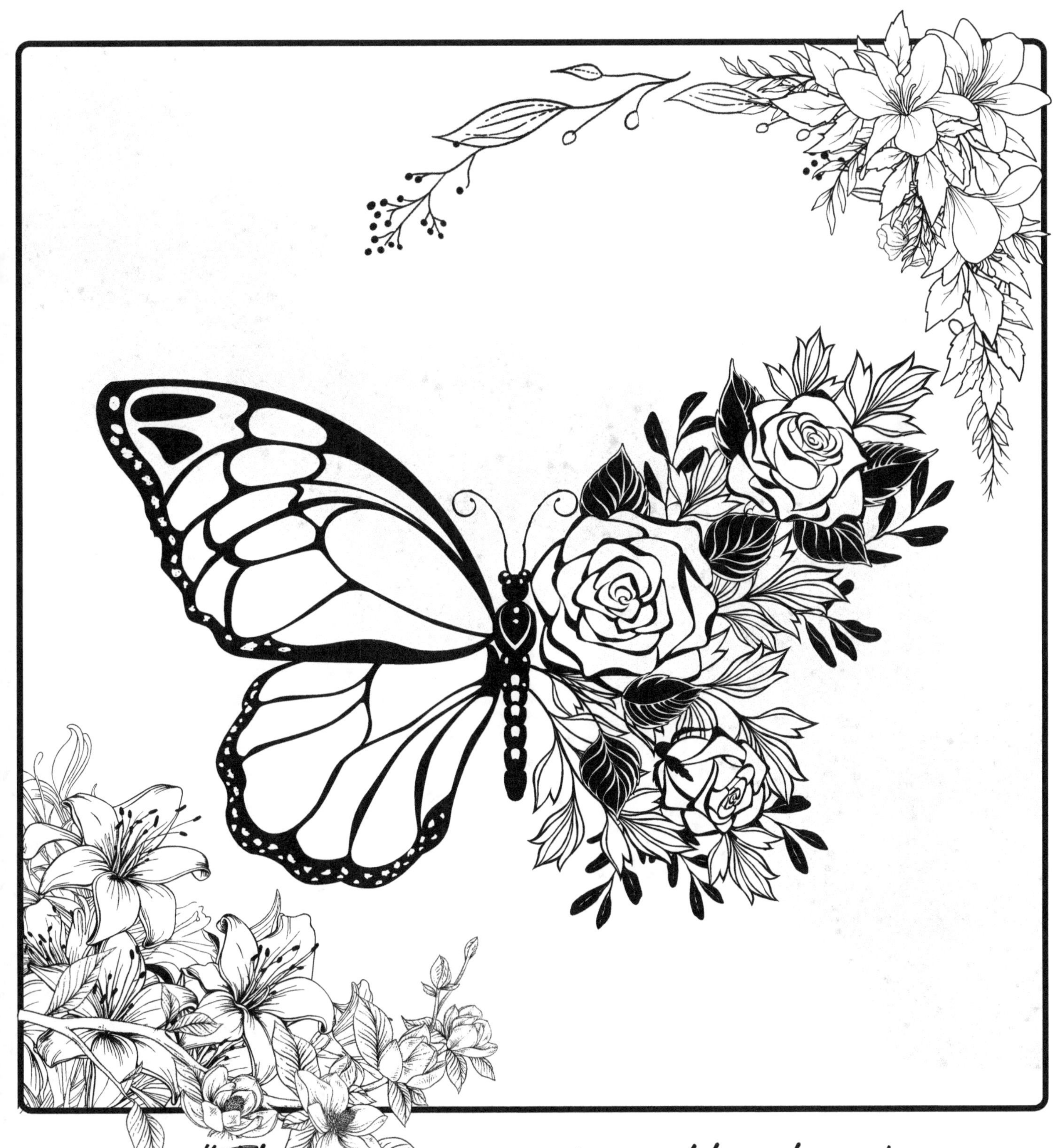

"The journey of motherhood
is filled with joy."

Growing Together

"Connect with other expectant mothers.
Sharing experiences can be comforting and helpful."

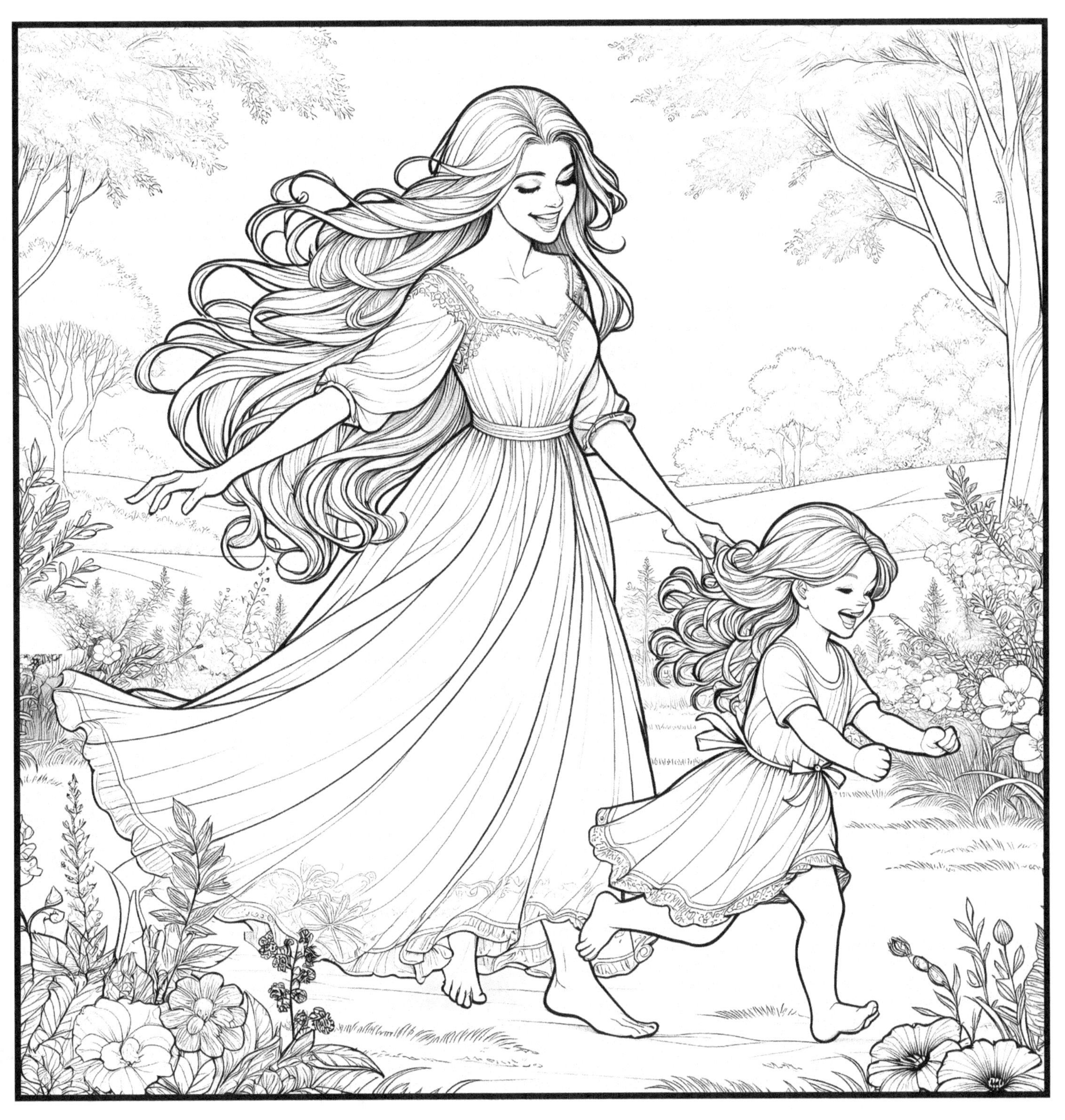

"Celebrate the little moments
along the way."

Growing Together

"This journey is filled with hope and happiness.
Embrace each moment with love and joy."

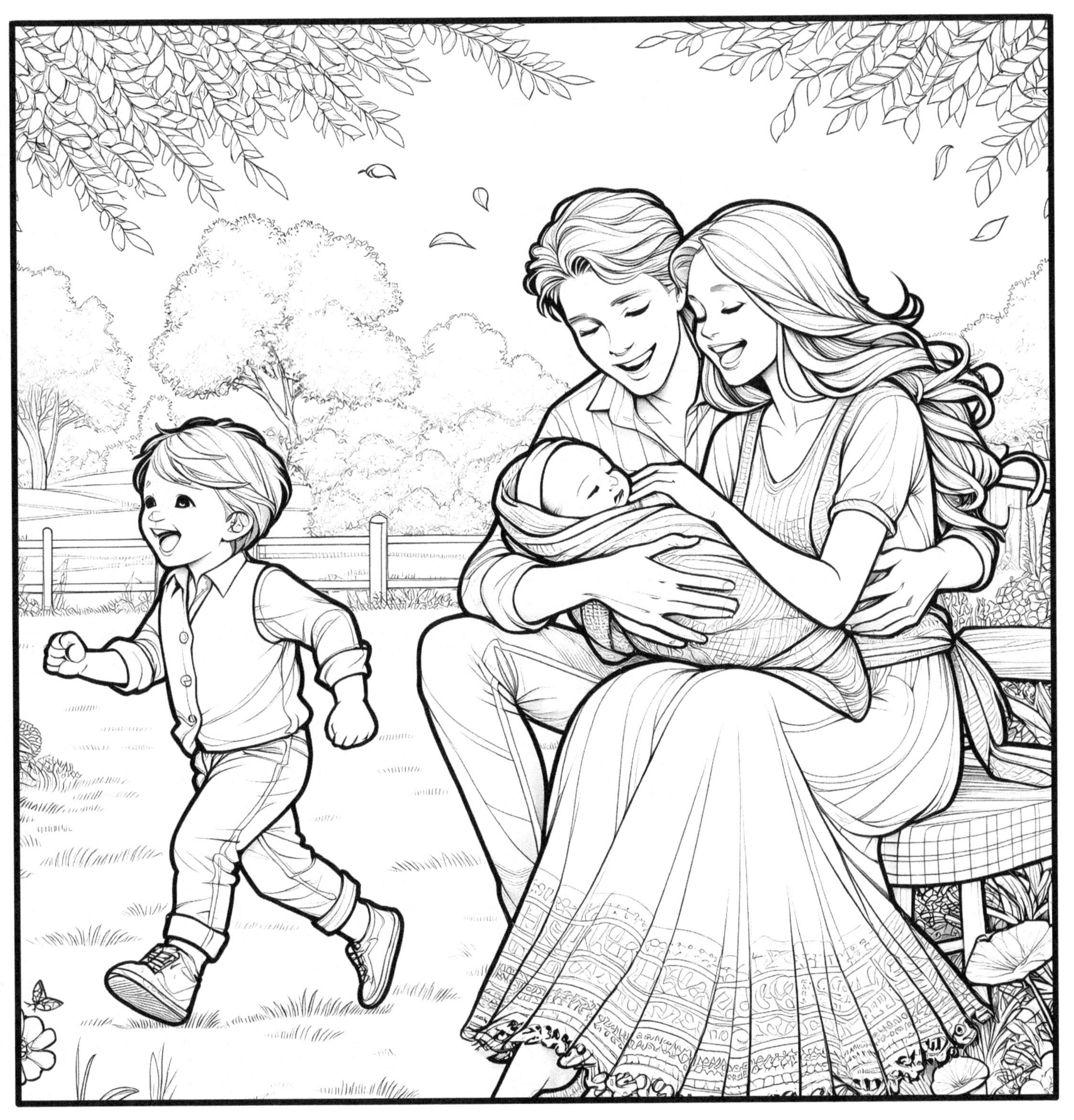

*"Your heart is growing along
with your baby."*

Growing Together

"Do things that make you happy.
A joyful mom makes a joyful baby."

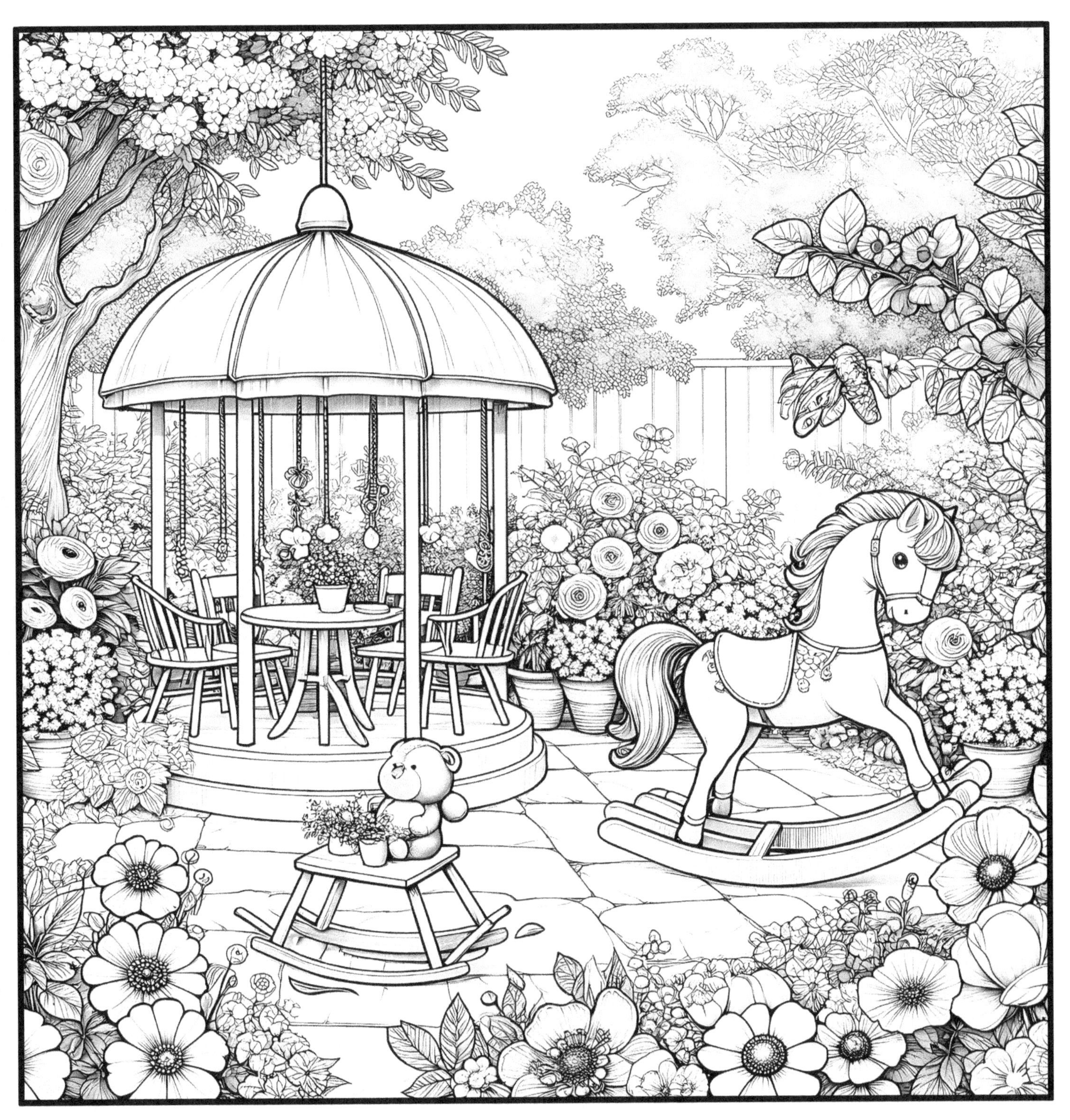

You are nurturing a miracle.

Growing Together

"Feeling your baby's heartbeat is a magical moment.
Enjoy this special connection.
Every kick and movement is a sign
that your baby is growing strong and healthy.
Celebrate these milestones."

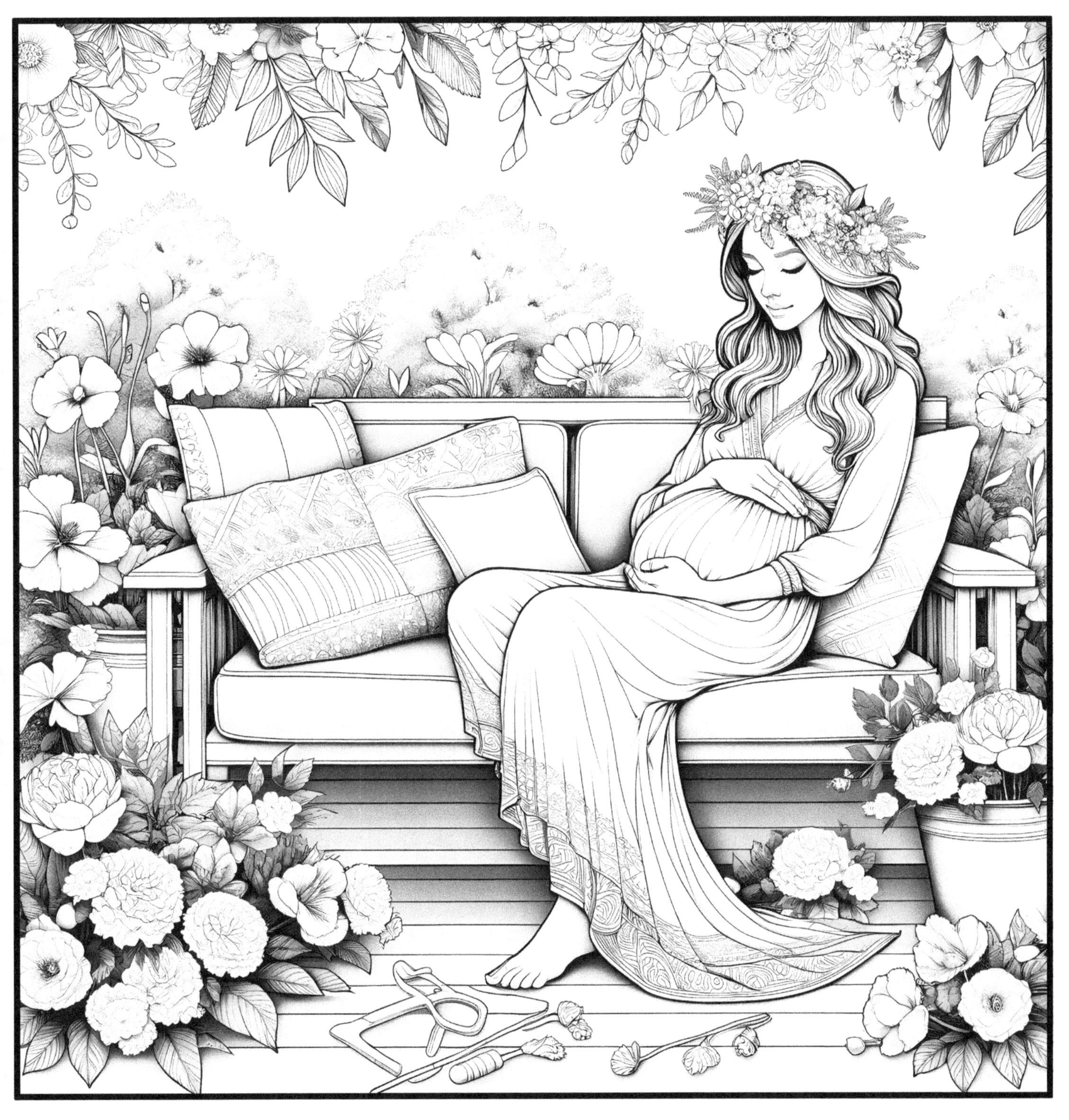

"Every heartbeat is a step closer
to meeting your baby."

Growing
Together

"A walk in the park can be refreshing.
Imagine your baby enjoying the gentle sway as you walk."

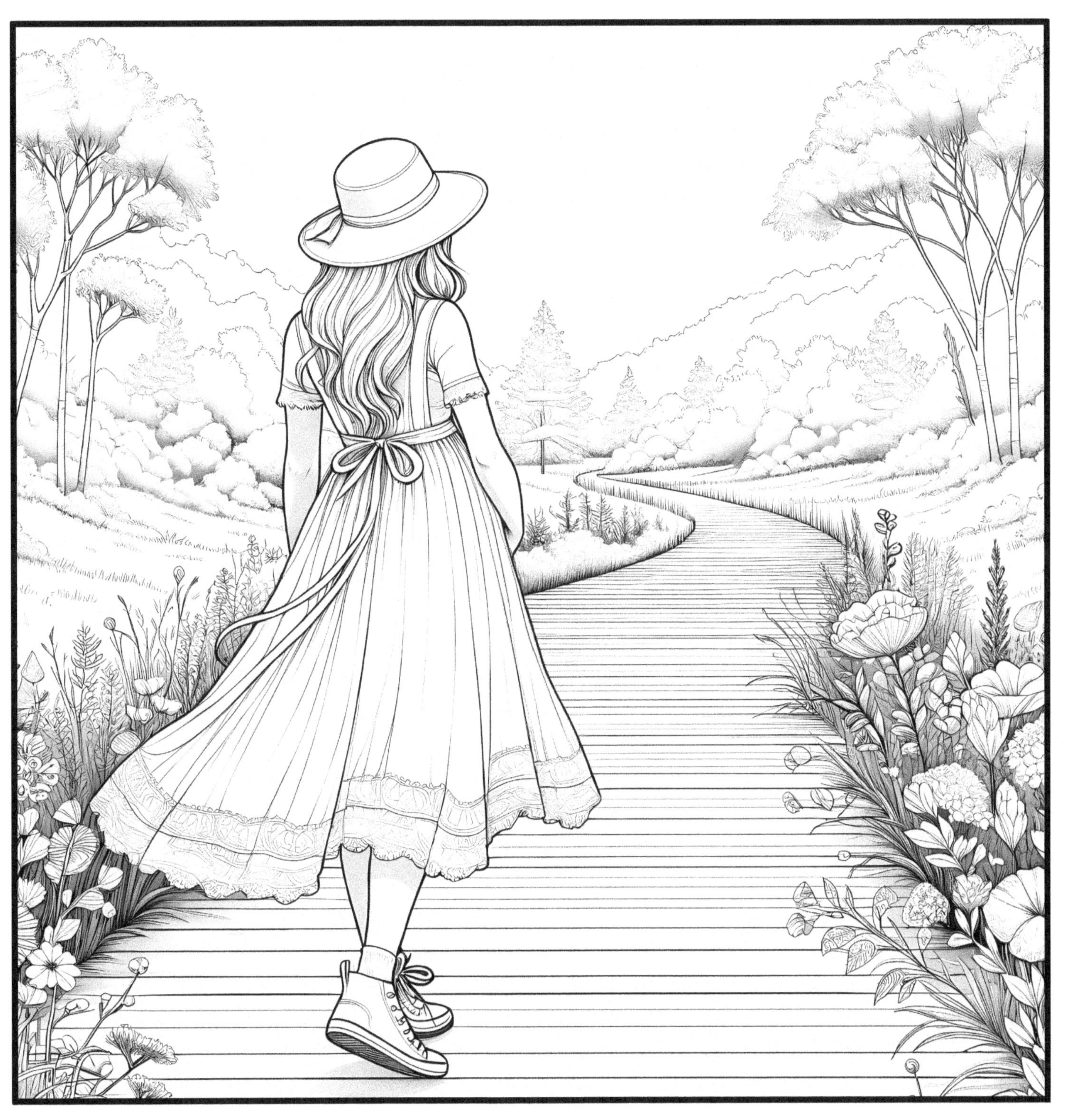

"Embrace the journey,
it is uniquely yours."

Growing Together

"Every change in your body is a sign of your baby's growth.
Embrace these beautiful changes."

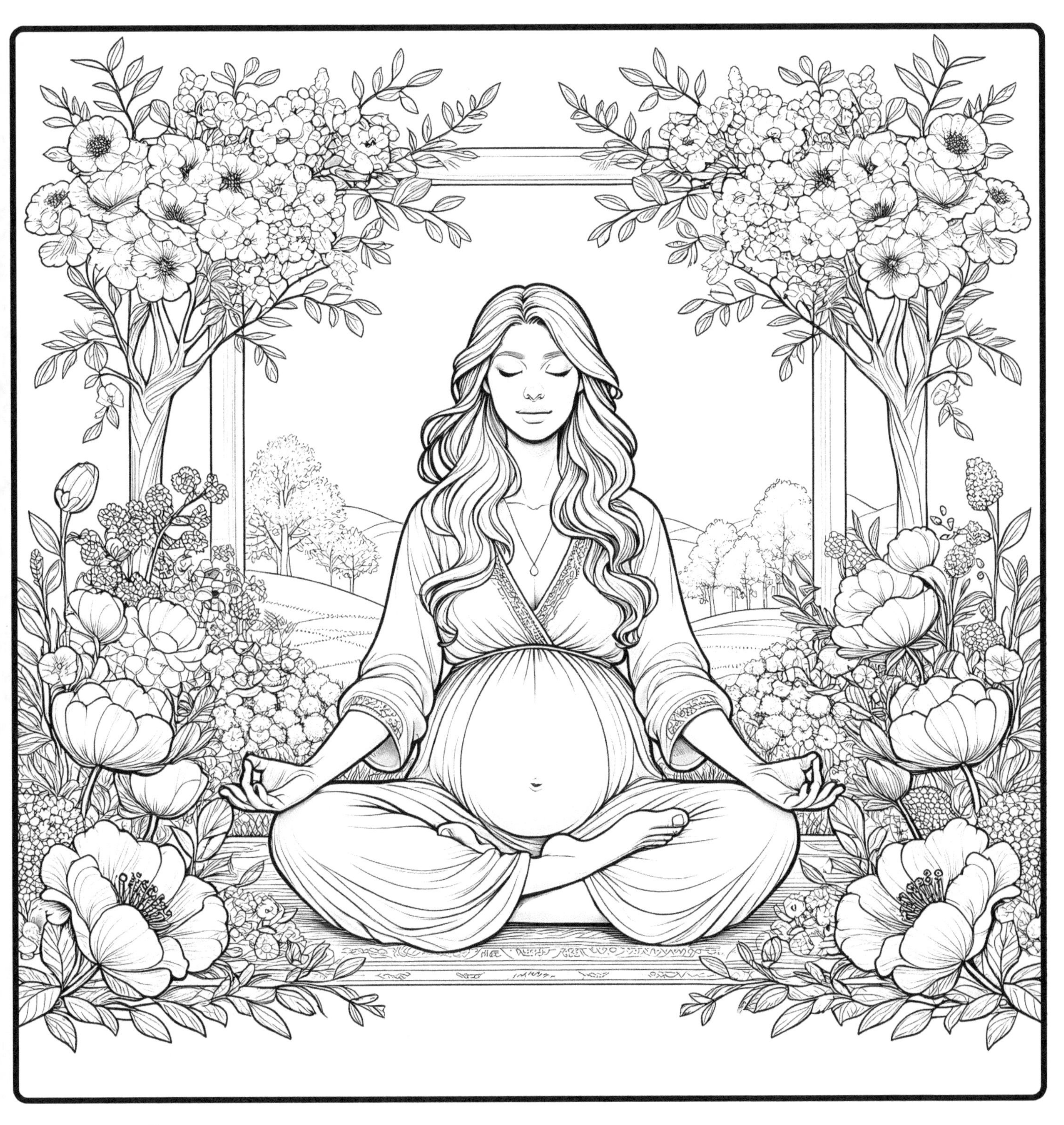

You are amazing in every way.

Growing
Together

"Water is soothing.
Spend time by a lake or take a warm bath to relax."

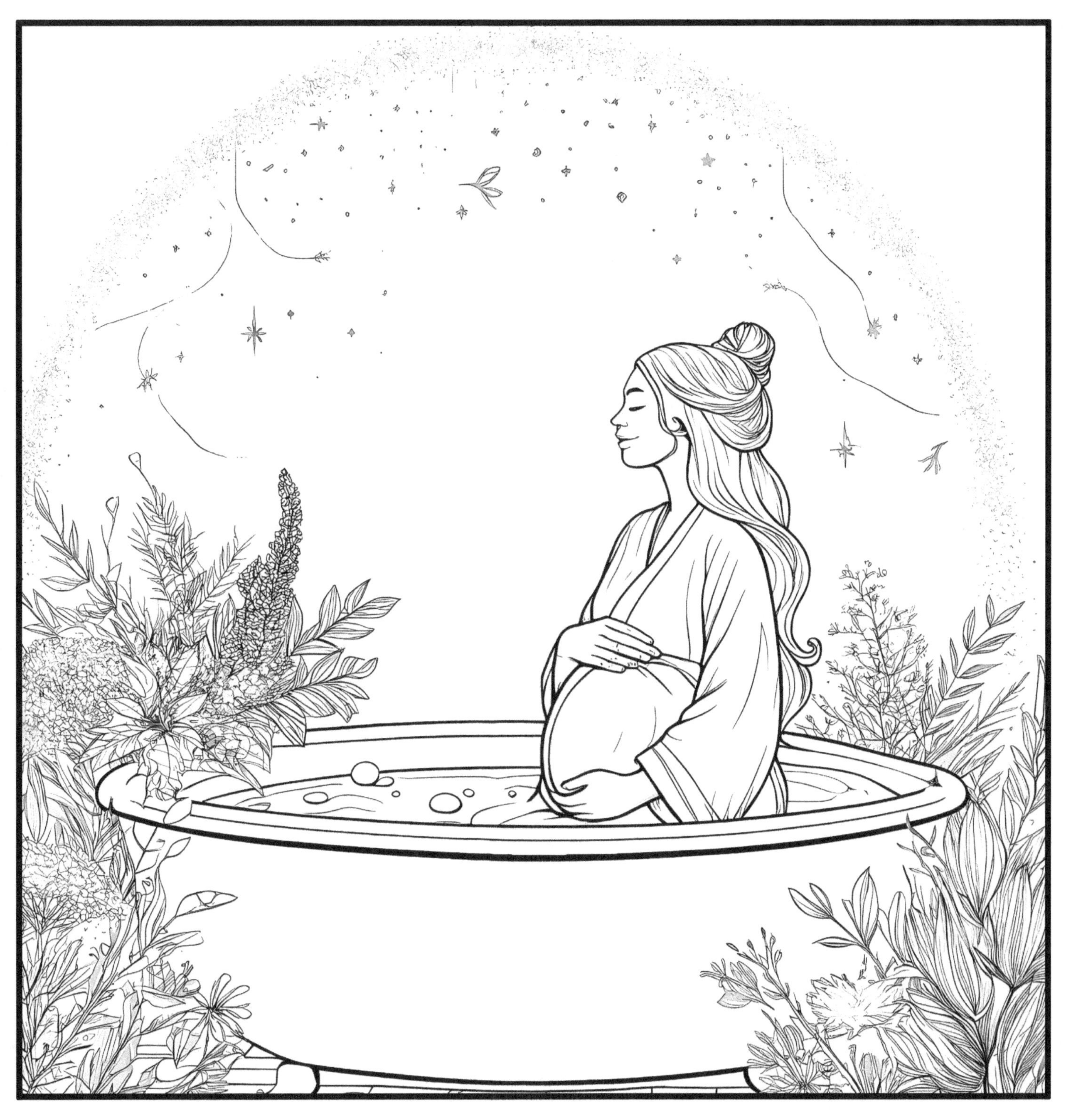

"*Your love creates a world of wonder.*"

Growing Together

"Pregnancy is a journey filled with hope and happiness.
Every step you take is preparing you to be a wonderful mother.
May you find joy in every moment of this journey,
and be ready to embrace the new chapter of your life
with love and hope."

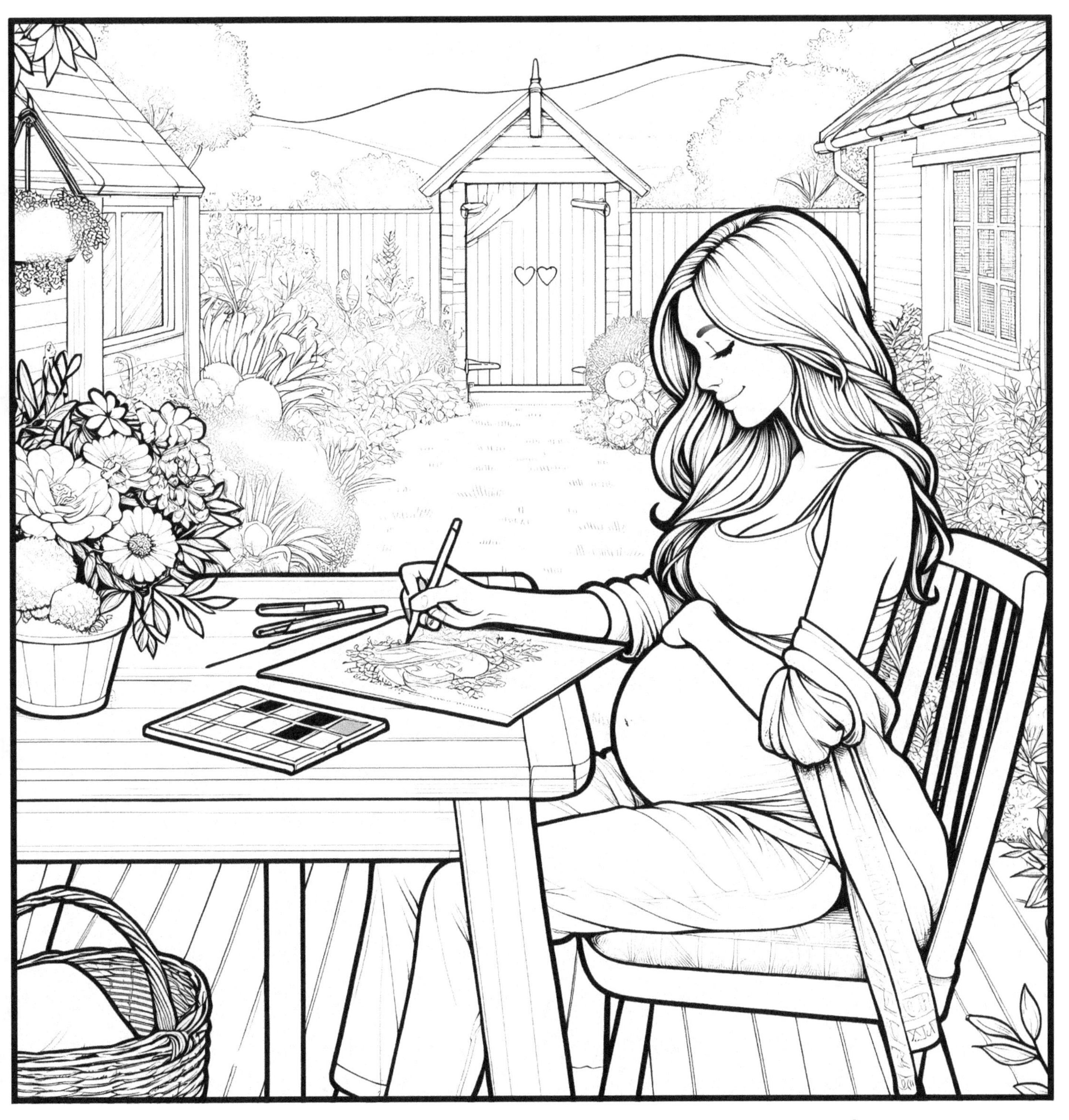

"This journey is filled with hope and happiness."

Next up
"Blossoming Moments"
A Coloring Book for the Second Trimester

Dear friend,

Thank you for spending this special journey with me during your important first trimester. I hope these coloring pages have brought you joy and peace, and that your beautiful artwork has created lovely memories and feelings as you await your little one.

Remember to take care of yourself and rest whenever you need to. Don't pressure yourself, your health and happiness are very important to me.

If you enjoyed this coloring book, I have another one to recommend "Blossoming Moments" A Coloring Book for the Second Trimester. We can continue sharing happiness and wonderful memories together during your second trimester.

Wishing you wonderful times filled with love. If there's anything I can do to help you through this journey, please let me know.

With love and care,
KB Klinsukont